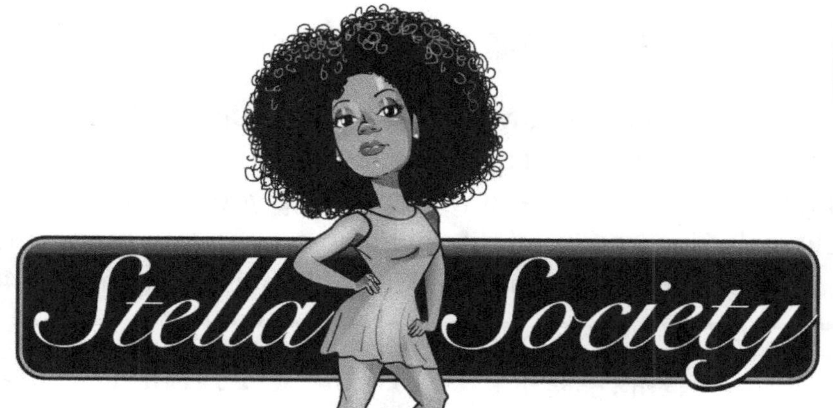

Thank you for participating in the Stella Project 2.0, a 40 day fitness confidence and nutrition challenge. If you purchased this journal and you are not a member of the Stella Project, no worries. You can find us at stellasocietyacademy dot com, or just use it on your own 40 day fitness journey.

Always consult a physician before beginning an exercise program.

How to use your journal

Journaling has many benefits especially when tracking progress. Recording your thoughts before training can help you better understand why a workout did or didn't go too well. Recalling the times you eat and what can help you combat unnecessary cravings. Journaling also increases self-discipline, improves your mood and boost comprehension. Please use this journal to aid in your goals through your 40 days.

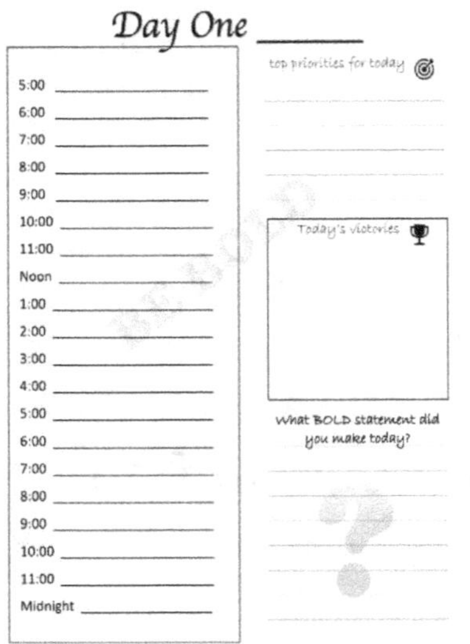

Use this page to record your daily schedule, meals, training, meetings, etc. Make sure you put the date. List your top priorities hat must be completed that day. Record your victories, like drinking all your water and reflect on the daily bestellatude

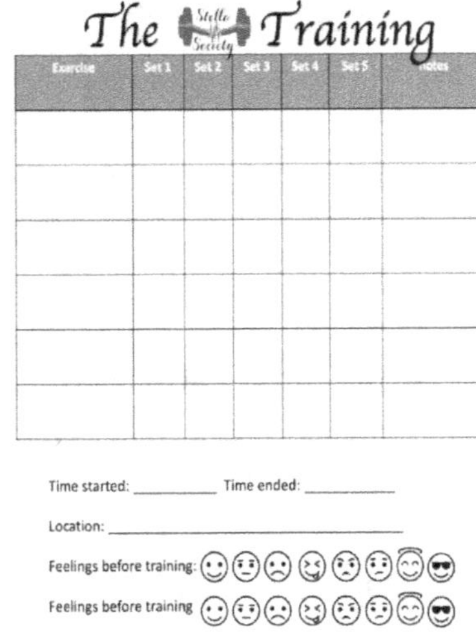

Use this page to record your training sessions. Write them down ahead of time and watch the video in case you have questions. Put the time your started and completed the training as well as how you felt before and after. Leave a note as to why you felt a certain before the training. This could effect how it went.

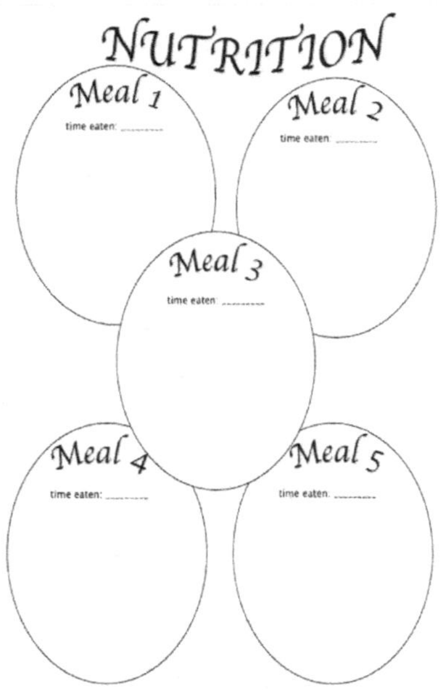

Use this page to record your meals and the time you ate them. This is important especially when tracking your progress. Try to eat your meals at the same time each day. Get your machine on a schedule so it knows how to operate its fuel.

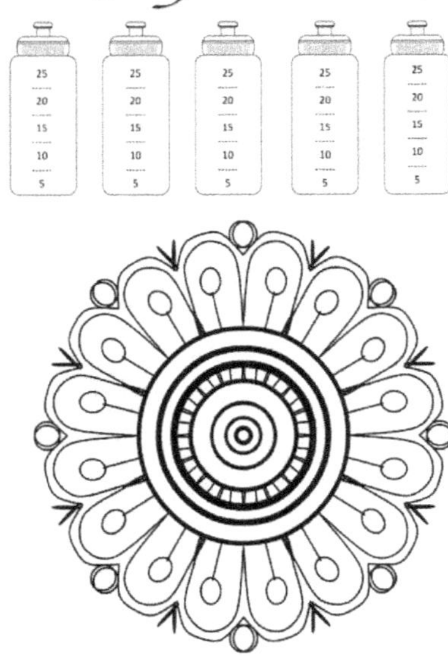

Use this page to record your water intake. Color the bottles as you complete each one. Also each hydration page has a mandala graphic to color. Coloring is a form of meditation. Choose to color this instead of reaching for something to snack on that's not you're your meal plan.

R.O.S.E.S GOAL

Rationale – why are you participating in this 40 day challenge?

____

____

Objective – what do you look to accomplish during the 40 days? What is the end game, goal?

____

____

Strategy – how will you go about completing your objective? What actions will you take.

____

____

Evaluation – how and when will you evaluate you progress? Will you use inches, weight, look, or clothes?

____

____

Schedule – create a schedule for the next 40 days. Include anything that will get in the way of your goal and find a work around.

____

____

Measurements

DATE: ___________

Weight: _______

Neck _______

Shoulders _______

Chest _______

Bicep / upper arm left ________ right _______

Forearm left ________ right _______

Waist _______

Hips _______

Thighs left ________ right _______

Calf left ________ right _______

**Only I Can Change My Life,
No One Can Do It For Me**

Day One _______

5:00 _______________________

6:00 _______________________

7:00 _______________________

8:00 _______________________

9:00 _______________________

10:00 ______________________

11:00 ______________________

Noon _______________________

1:00 _______________________

2:00 _______________________

3:00 _______________________

4:00 _______________________

5:00 _______________________

6:00 _______________________

7:00 _______________________

8:00 _______________________

9:00 _______________________

10:00 ______________________

11:00 ______________________

Midnight ___________________

top priorities for today

____

____

____

____

Today's victories 🏆

What BOLD statement did you make today?

____

____

____

____

____

____

The Training

Exercise	Set 1	Set 2	Set 3	Set 4	Set 5	notes

Time started: _____________ Time ended: _______________

Location: ____

Feelings before training:

Feelings after training

NUTRITION

Meal 1
time eaten: _________

Meal 2
time eaten: _________

Meal 3
time eaten: _________

Meal 4
time eaten: _________

Meal 5
time eaten: _________

Hydration

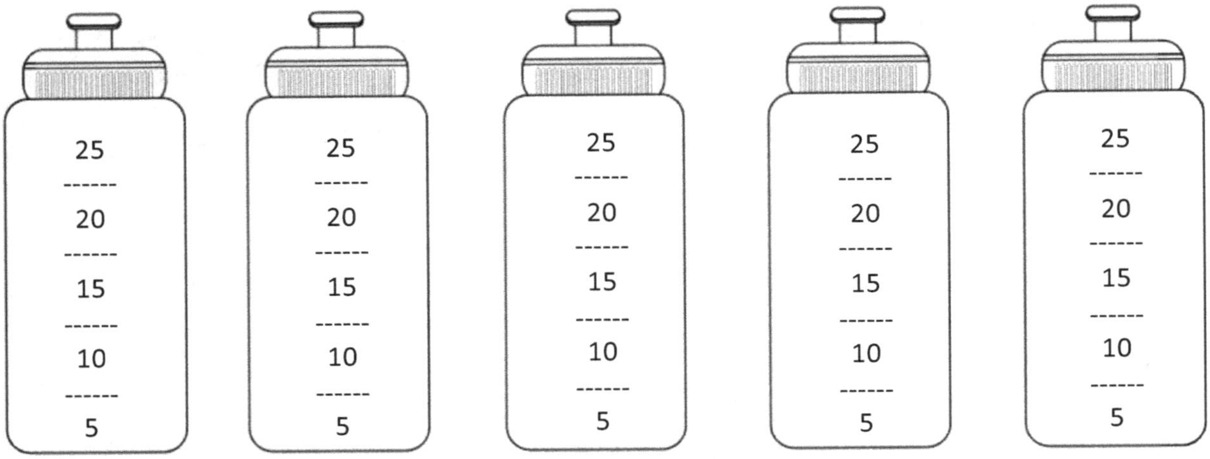

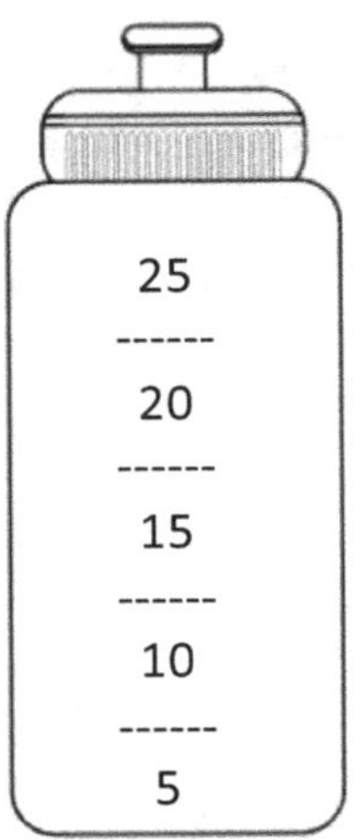
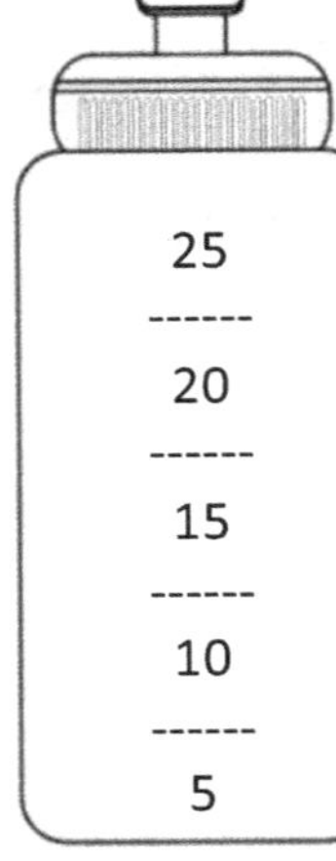
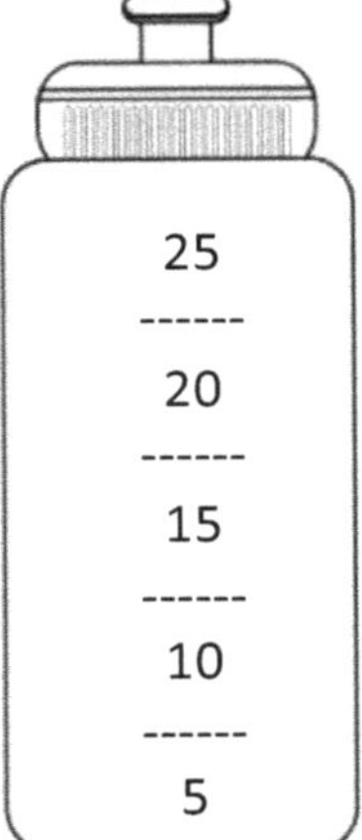
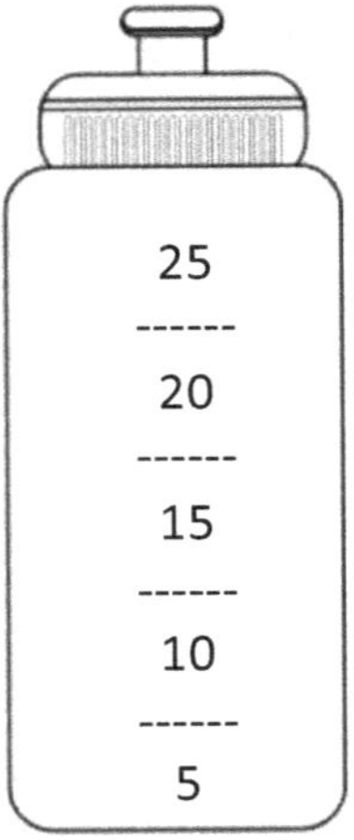

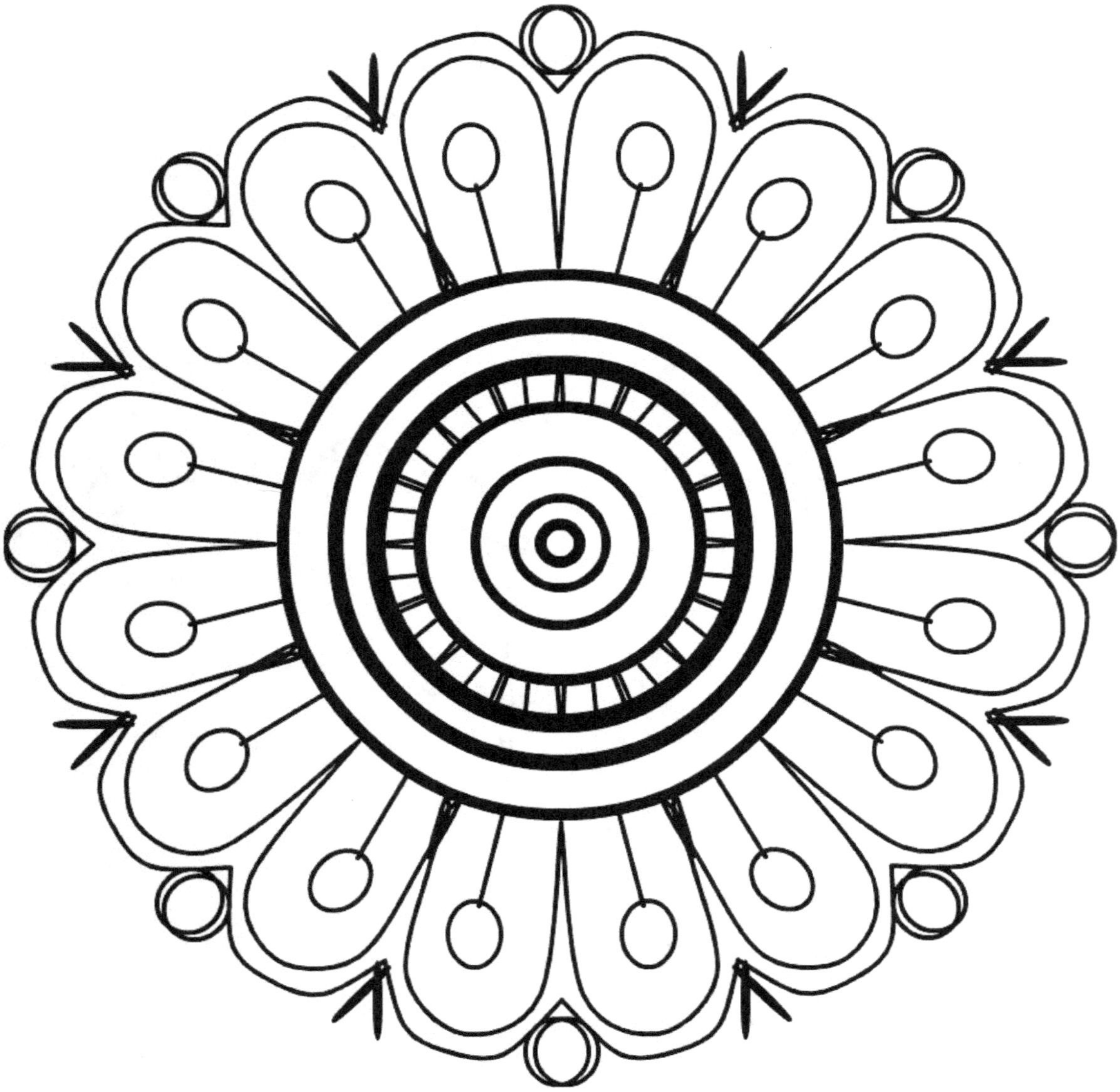

Day Two _______

5:00 _____________	top priorities for today 🎯
6:00 _____________	
7:00 _____________	_____________
8:00 _____________	_____________
9:00 _____________	_____________
10:00 _____________	_____________
11:00 _____________	

5:00 _______________________

6:00 _______________________

7:00 _______________________

8:00 _______________________

9:00 _______________________

10:00 ______________________

11:00 ______________________

Noon _______________________

1:00 _______________________

2:00 _______________________

3:00 _______________________

4:00 _______________________

5:00 _______________________

6:00 _______________________

7:00 _______________________

8:00 _______________________

9:00 _______________________

10:00 ______________________

11:00 ______________________

Midnight ___________________

top priorities for today 🎯

____

____

____

____

Today's victories 🏆

What is one thing that makes you unique??

____

____

____

____

____

The Training

Exercise	Set 1	Set 2	Set 3	Set 4	Set 5	notes

Time started: _____________ Time ended: _____________

Location: ____

Feelings before training: 🙂 😐 ☹️ 😜 😠 😕 😇 😎

Feelings after training 🙂 😐 ☹️ 😜 😠 😕 😇 😎

NUTRITION

Meal 1

time eaten: _________

Meal 2

time eaten: _________

Meal 3

time eaten: _________

Meal 4

time eaten: _________

Meal 5

time eaten: _________

Hydration

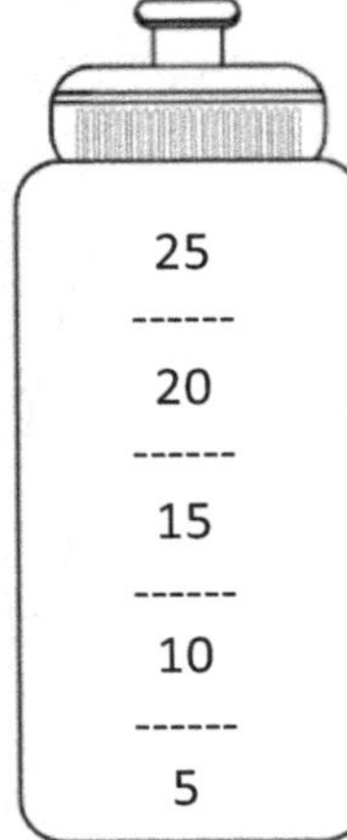

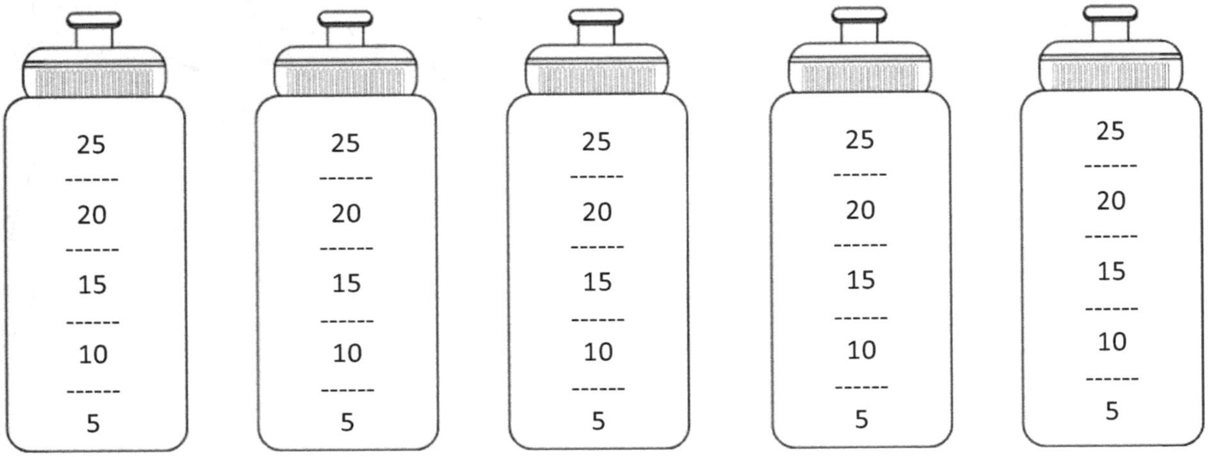

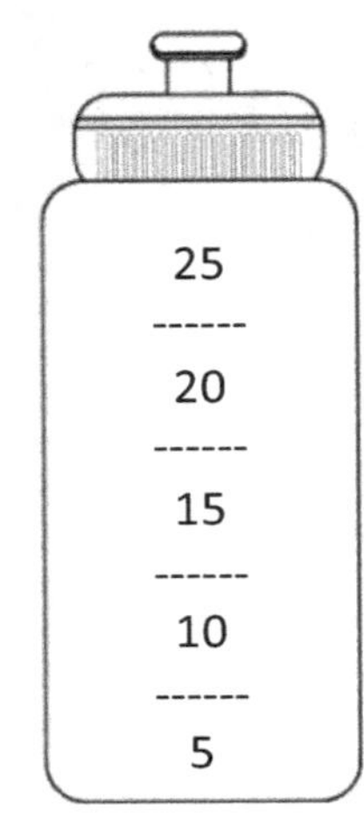

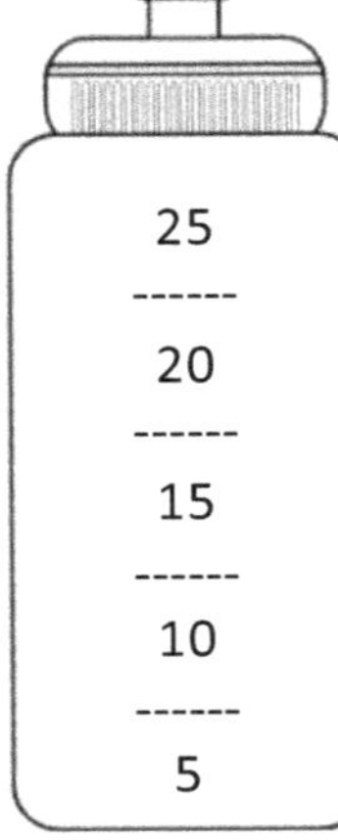

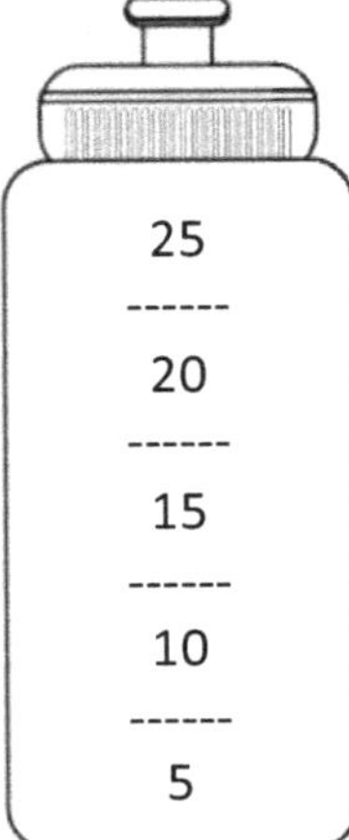

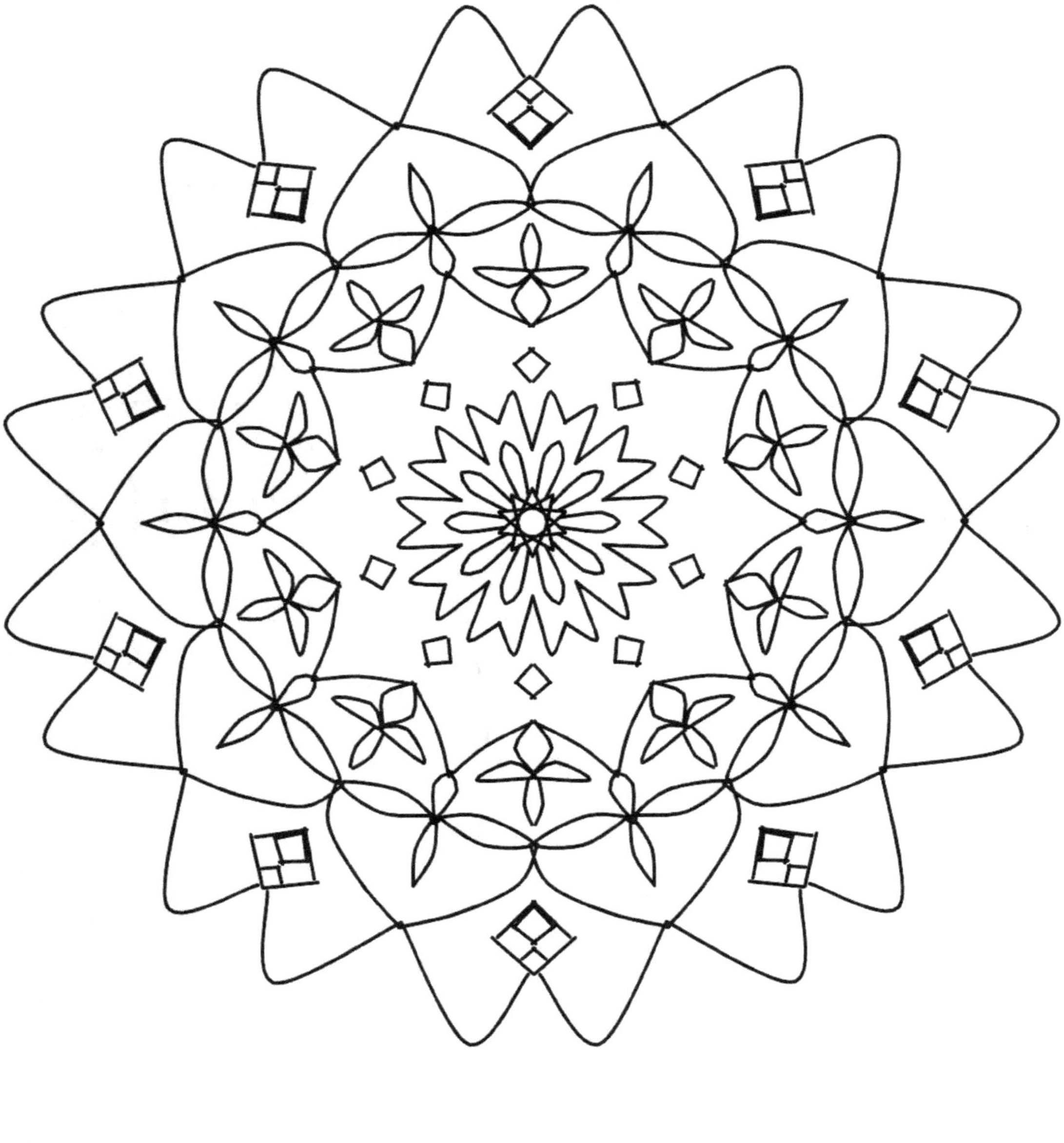

Day Three _______

5:00 ____________	

5:00 ________________

6:00 ________________

7:00 ________________

8:00 ________________

9:00 ________________

10:00 ________________

11:00 ________________

Noon ________________

1:00 ________________

2:00 ________________

3:00 ________________

4:00 ________________

5:00 ________________

6:00 ________________

7:00 ________________

8:00 ________________

9:00 ________________

10:00 ________________

11:00 ________________

Midnight ________________

top priorities for today

____

____

____

____

Today's victories

What makes you brave?

____

____

____

____

____

____

The Training

Exercise	Set 1	Set 2	Set 3	Set 4	Set 5	notes

Time started: _______________   Time ended: _______________

Location: ____

Feelings before training:

Feelings after training

NUTRITION

Meal 1

time eaten: _________

Meal 2

time eaten: _________

Meal 3

time eaten: _________

Meal 4

time eaten: _________

Meal 5

time eaten: _________

Hydration

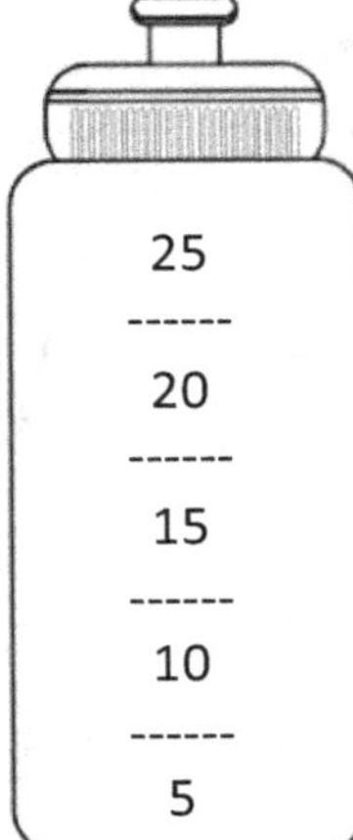

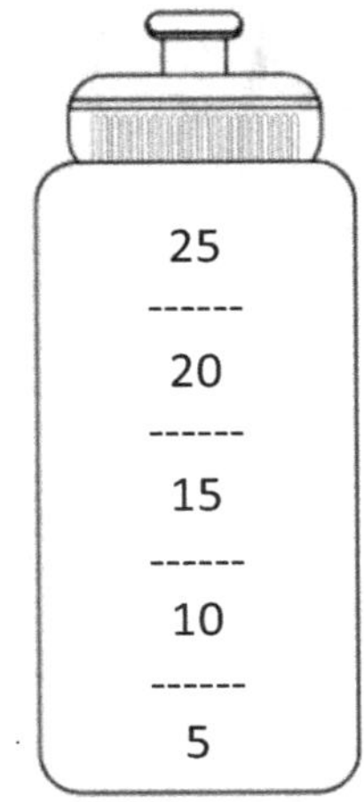

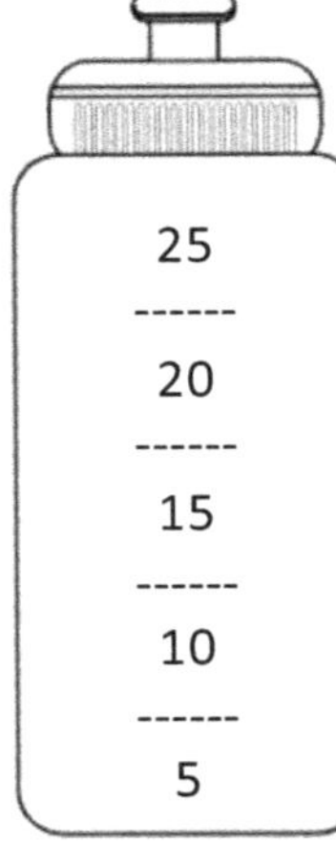

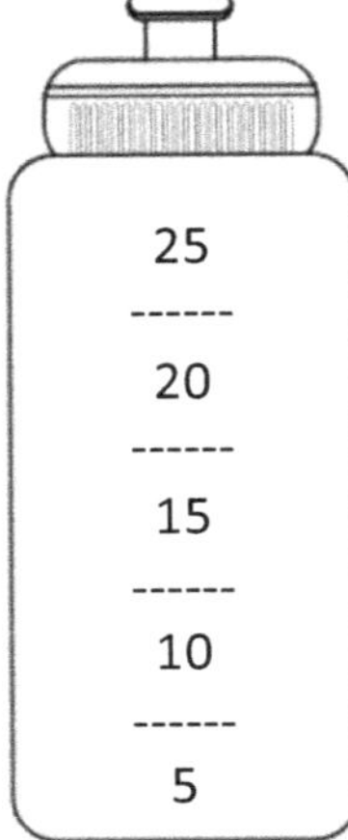

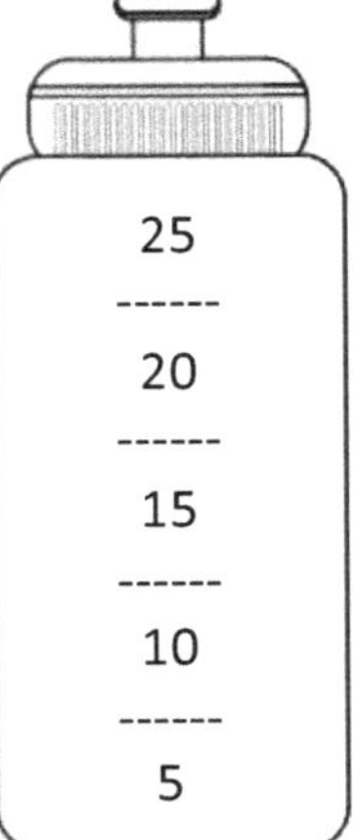

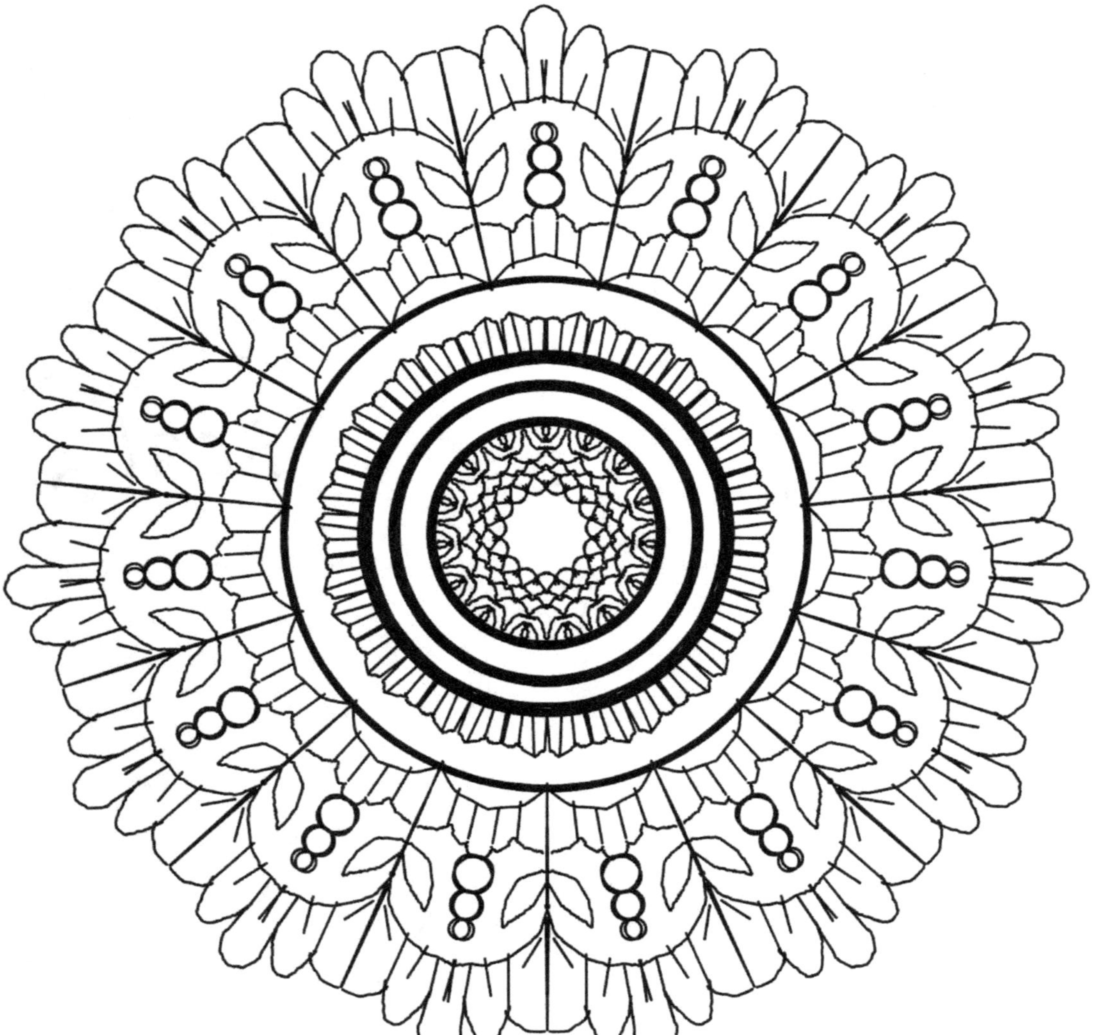

Day Four _______

<table>
<tr><td>

5:00 _______________________

6:00 _______________________

7:00 _______________________

8:00 _______________________

9:00 _______________________

10:00 ______________________

11:00 ______________________

Noon _______________________

1:00 _______________________

2:00 _______________________

3:00 _______________________

4:00 _______________________

5:00 _______________________

6:00 _______________________

7:00 _______________________

8:00 _______________________

9:00 _______________________

10:00 ______________________

11:00 ______________________

Midnight ___________________

</td><td>

top priorities for today 🎯

____

____

____

____

Today's victories 🏆

What did you commit to today that will make for a better tomorrow?

____

____

____

____

____

____

</td></tr>
</table>

The *Stella Society* Training

Exercise	Set 1	Set 2	Set 3	Set 4	Set 5	notes

Time started: _____________   Time ended: _______________

Location: ____

Feelings before training:

Feelings aftertraining

NUTRITION

Meal 1

time eaten: _________

Meal 2

time eaten: _________

Meal 3

time eaten: _________

Meal 4

time eaten: _________

Meal 5

time eaten: _________

Hydration

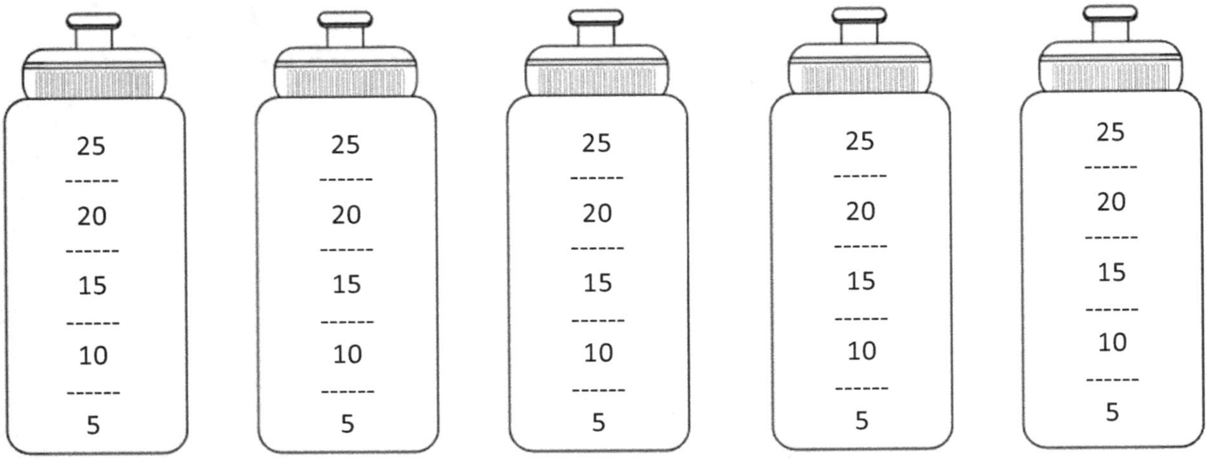

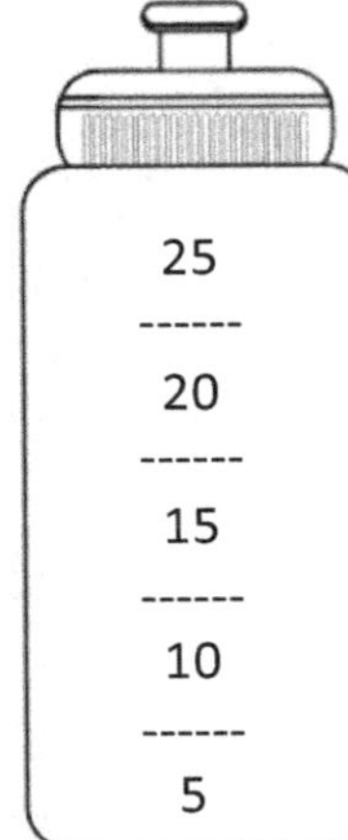
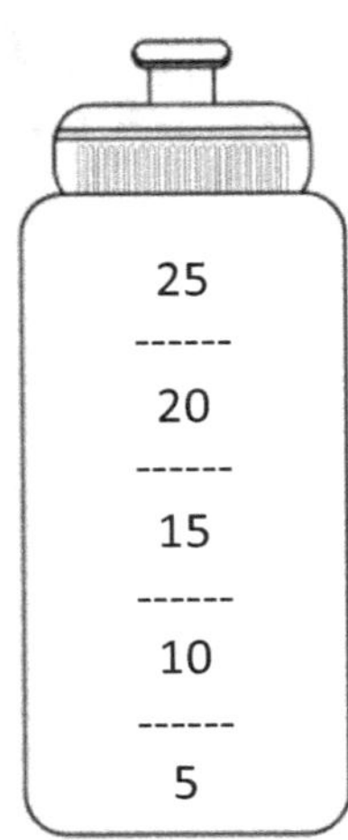
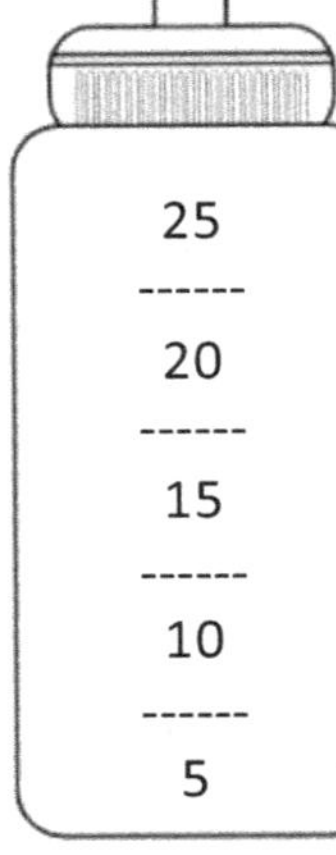
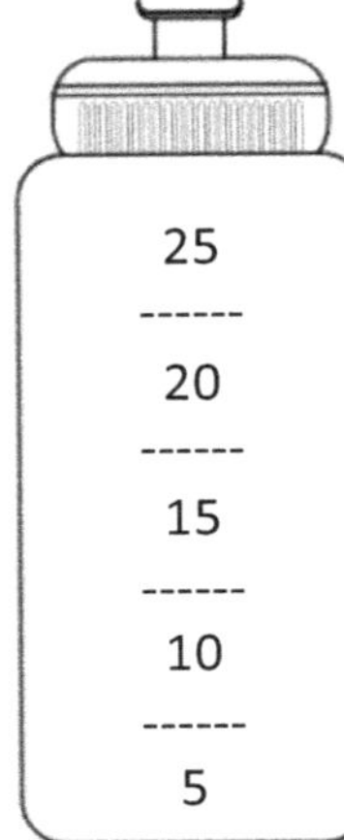
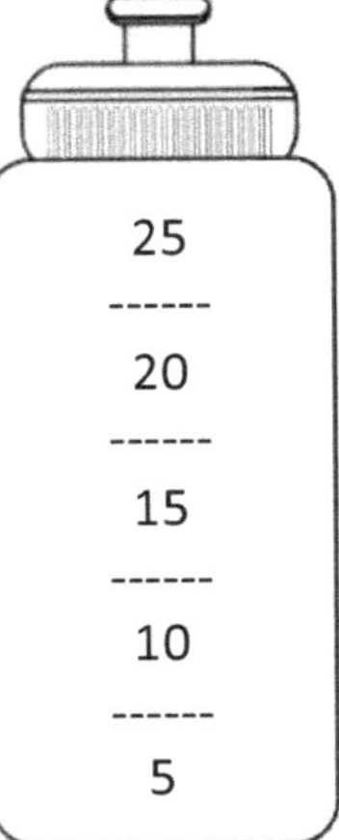

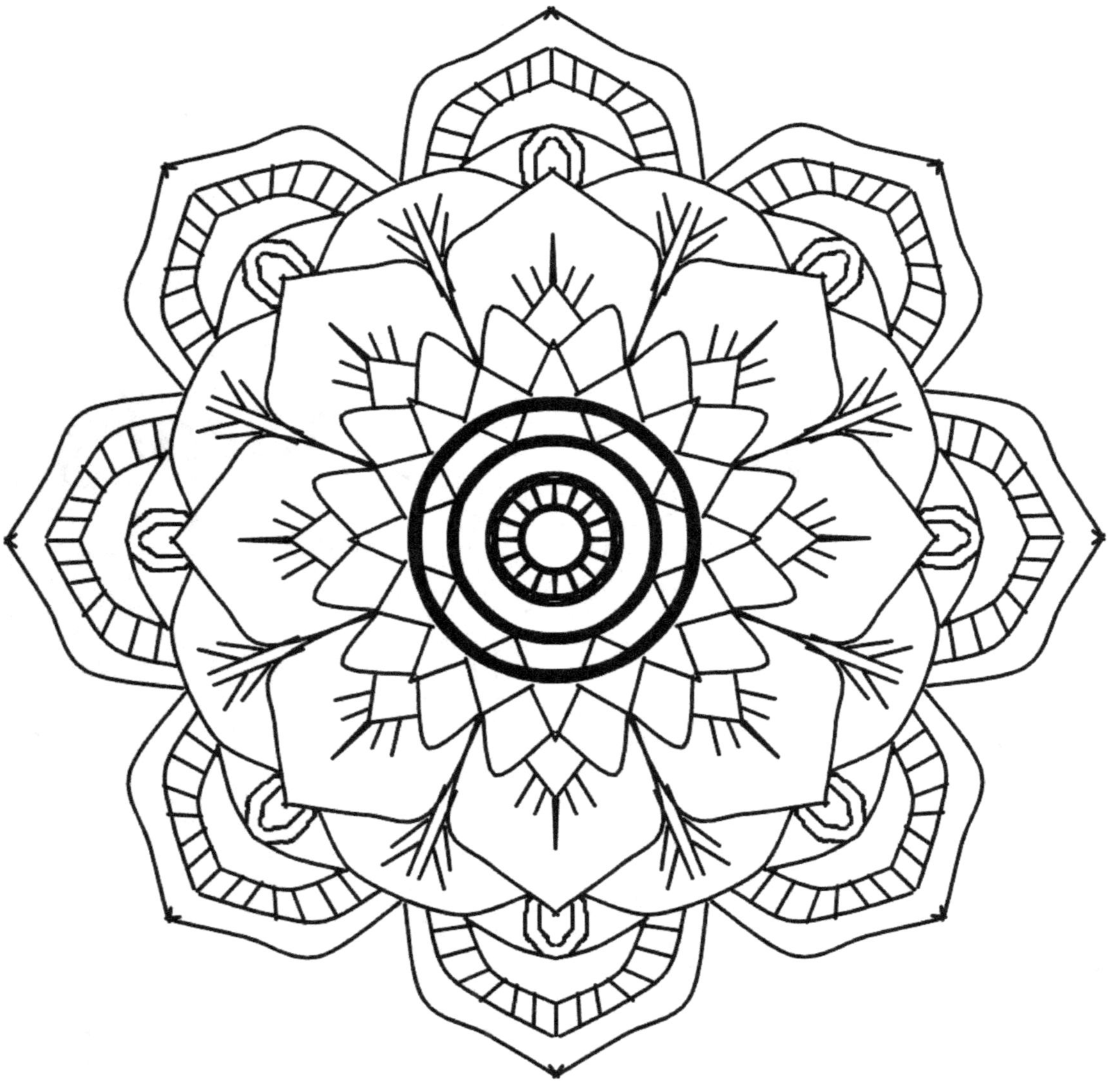

Day Five _______

5:00 _______________	top priorities for today 🎯
6:00 _______________	_______________
7:00 _______________	_______________
8:00 _______________	_______________
9:00 _______________	_______________
10:00 ______________	
11:00 ______________	**Today's victories** 🏆
Noon _______________	
1:00 _______________	
2:00 _______________	
3:00 _______________	
4:00 _______________	
5:00 _______________	Who is the wisest person you know?
6:00 _______________	Talk to them today.
7:00 _______________	_______________
8:00 _______________	_______________
9:00 _______________	_______________
10:00 ______________	_______________
11:00 ______________	_______________
Midnight ___________	_______________

The Training

Exercise	Set 1	Set 2	Set 3	Set 4	Set 5	notes

Time started: _______________ Time ended: _______________

Location: ____

Feelings before training:

Feelings after training

NUTRITION

Meal 1
time eaten: _________

Meal 2
time eaten: _________

Meal 3
time eaten: _________

Meal 4
time eaten: _________

Meal 5
time eaten: _________

Hydration

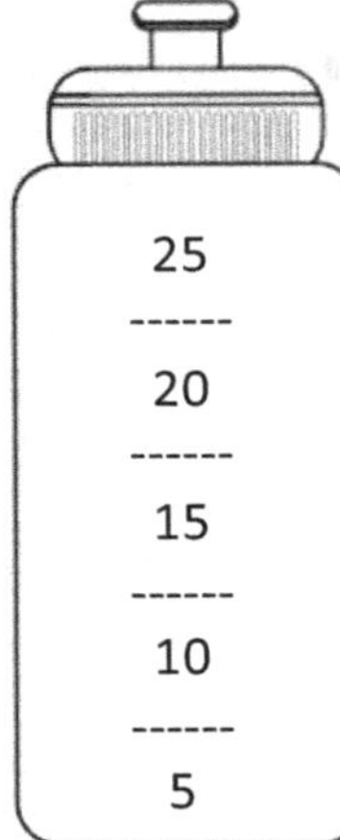
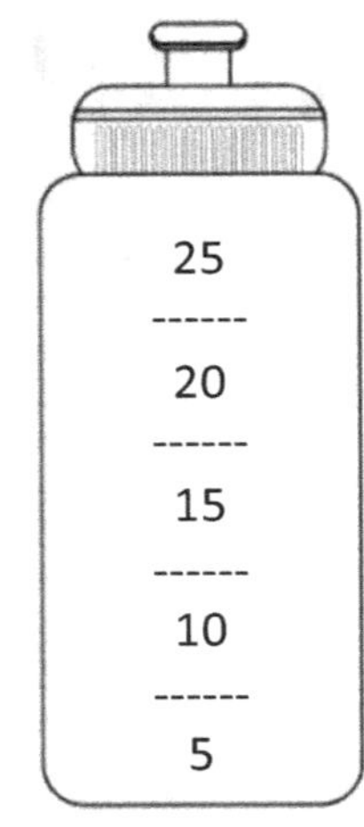
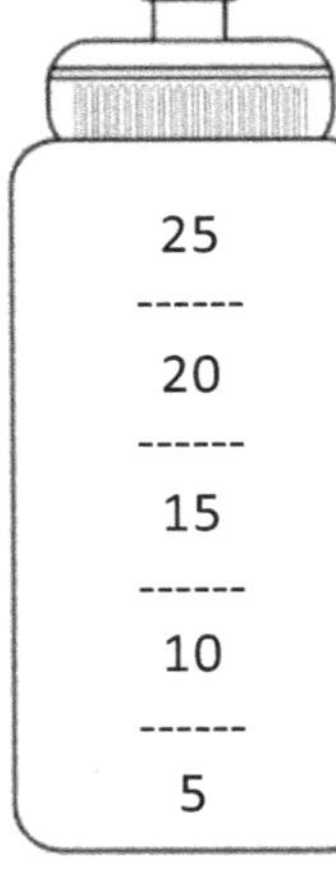
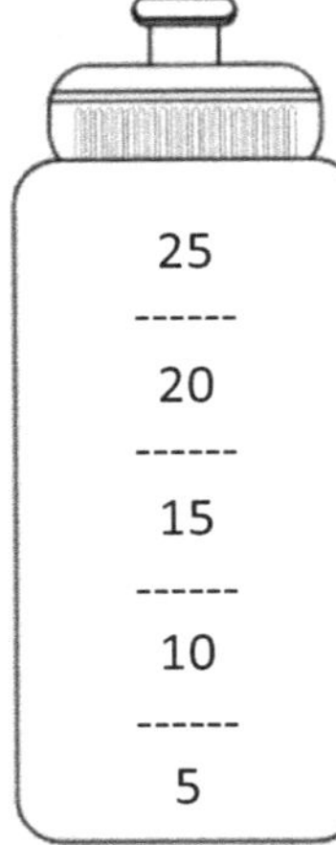
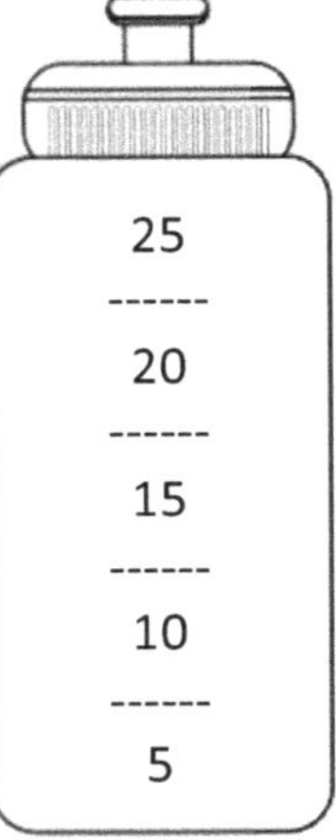

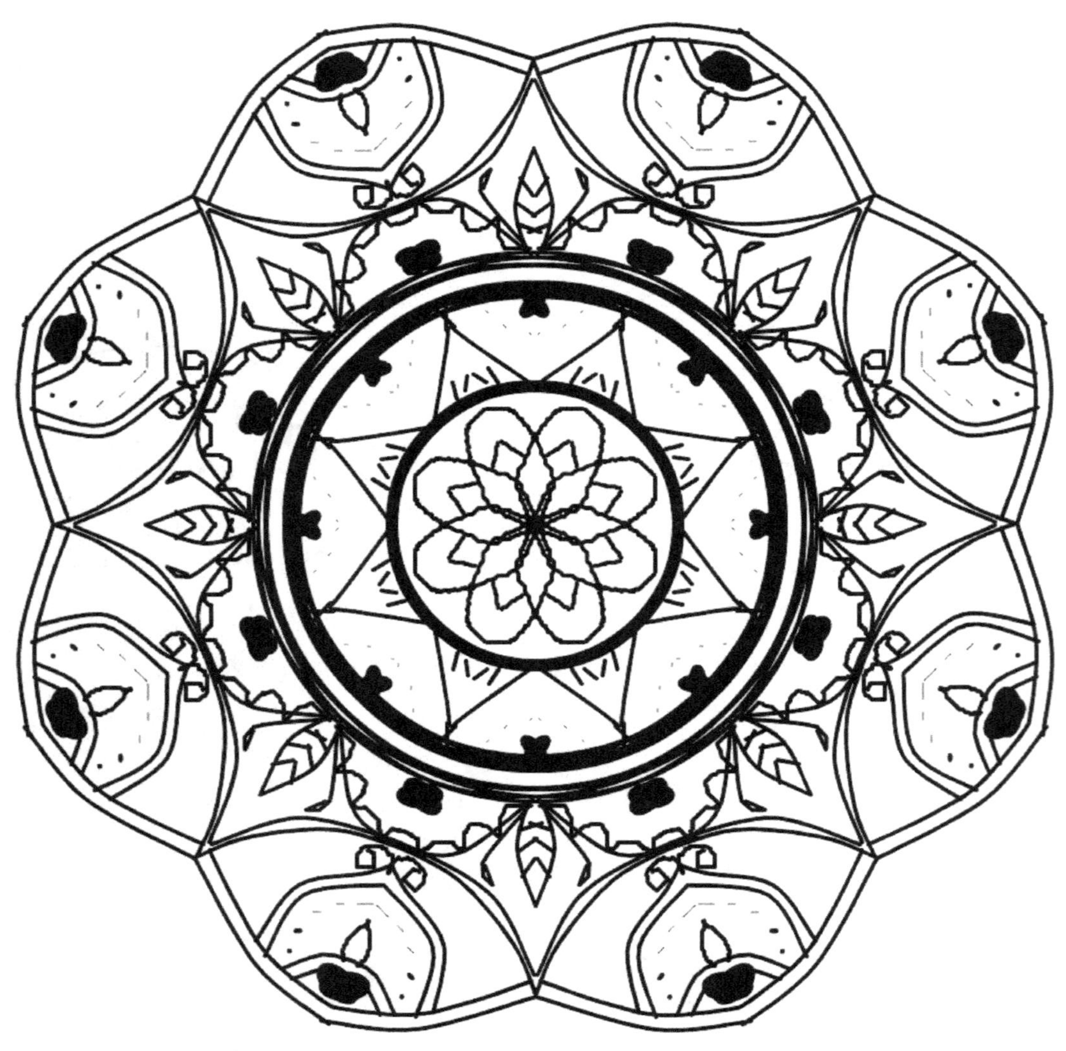

Day Six _______

5:00 _______________	

5:00 _______________
6:00 _______________
7:00 _______________
8:00 _______________
9:00 _______________
10:00 _______________
11:00 _______________
Noon _______________
1:00 _______________
2:00 _______________
3:00 _______________
4:00 _______________
5:00 _______________
6:00 _______________
7:00 _______________
8:00 _______________
9:00 _______________
10:00 _______________
11:00 _______________
Midnight _______________

top priorities for today 🎯

____
____
____
____

Today's victories 🏆

What is your biggest fear and how
do you get over it?

____
____
____
____
____
____

The Stella Society Training

Exercise	Set 1	Set 2	Set 3	Set 4	Set 5	notes

Time started: _____________   Time ended: _____________

Location: ____

Feelings before training:        

Feelings after training

NUTRITION

Meal 1
time eaten: _________

Meal 2
time eaten: _________

Meal 3
time eaten: _________

Meal 4
time eaten: _________

Meal 5
time eaten: _________

Hydration

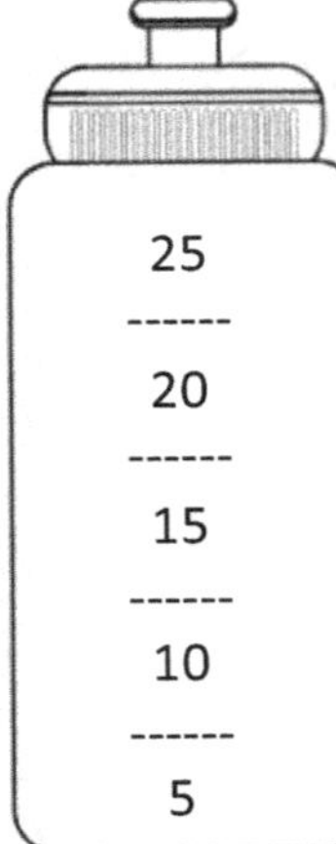

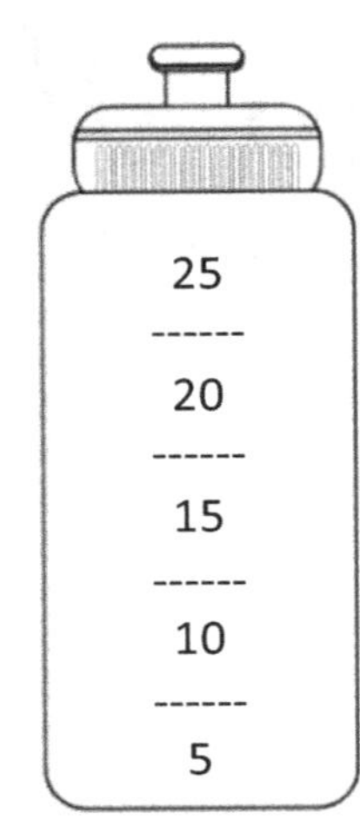

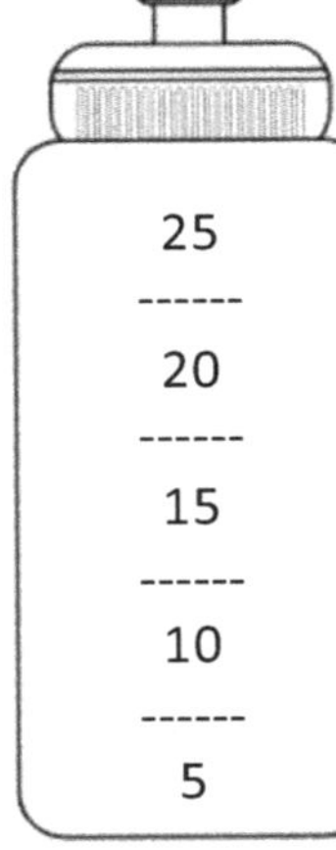

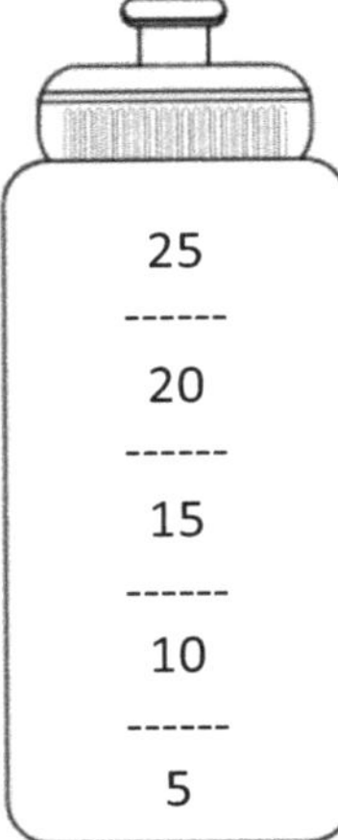

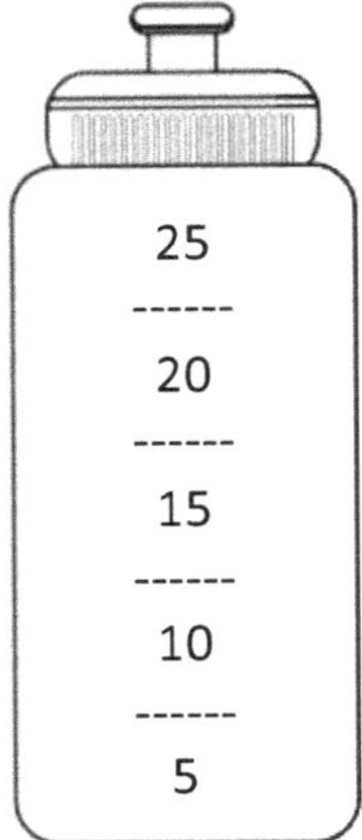

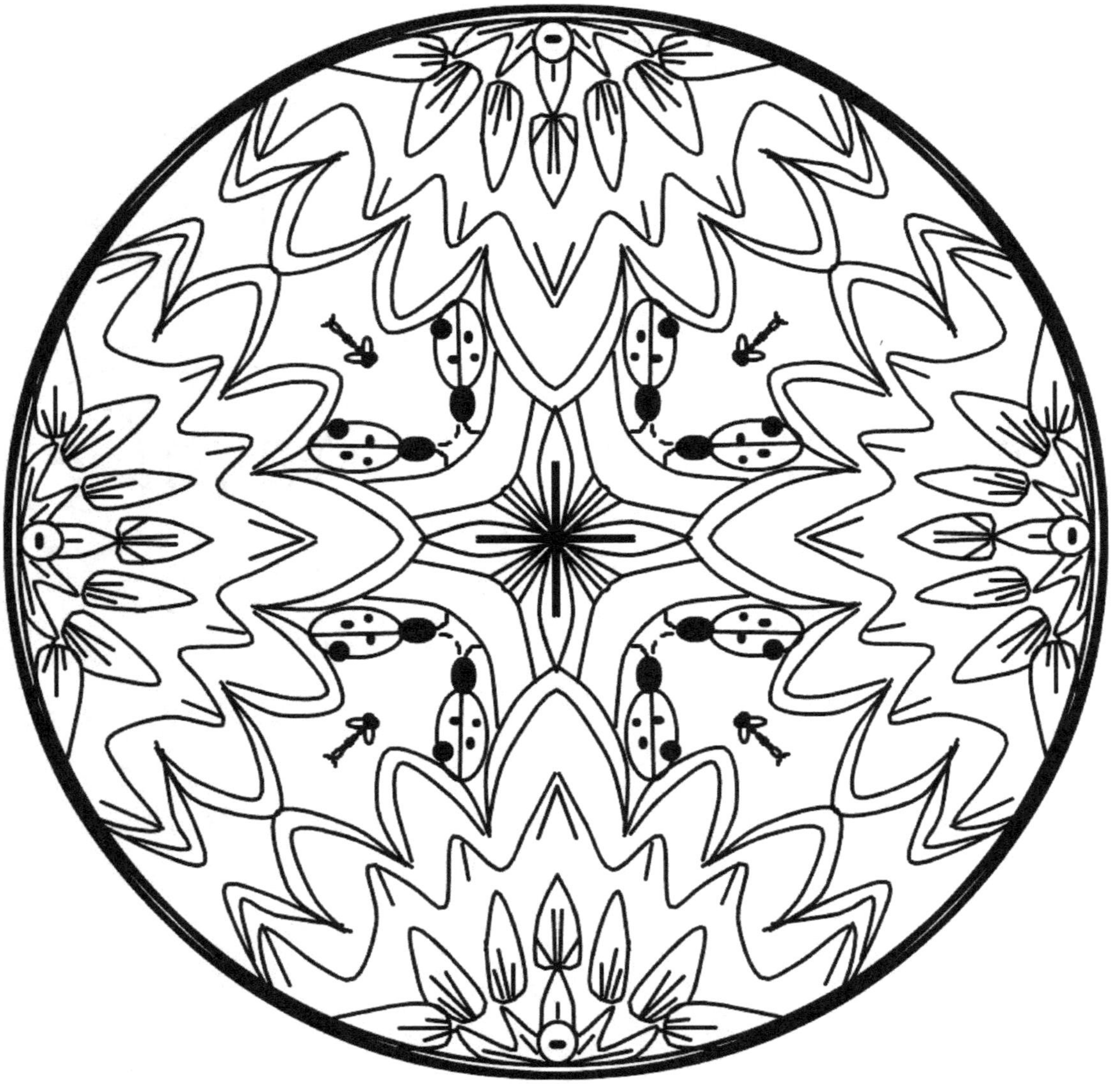

Day Seven ______

Time	
5:00	__________________
6:00	__________________
7:00	__________________
8:00	__________________
9:00	__________________
10:00	__________________
11:00	__________________
Noon	__________________
1:00	__________________
2:00	__________________
3:00	__________________
4:00	__________________
5:00	__________________
6:00	__________________
7:00	__________________
8:00	__________________
9:00	__________________
10:00	__________________
11:00	__________________
Midnight	__________________

top priorities for today

Today's victories

Where does your strength come from?

The Training

Exercise	Set 1	Set 2	Set 3	Set 4	Set 5	notes

Time started: _____________   Time ended: _____________

Location: ____

Feelings before training: 😊 😐 🙁 😜 😠 😕 😇 😎

Feelings after training 😊 😐 🙁 😜 😠 😕 😇 😎

NUTRITION

Meal 1

time eaten: _________

Meal 2

time eaten: _________

Meal 3

time eaten: _________

Meal 4

time eaten: _________

Meal 5

time eaten: _________

Hydration

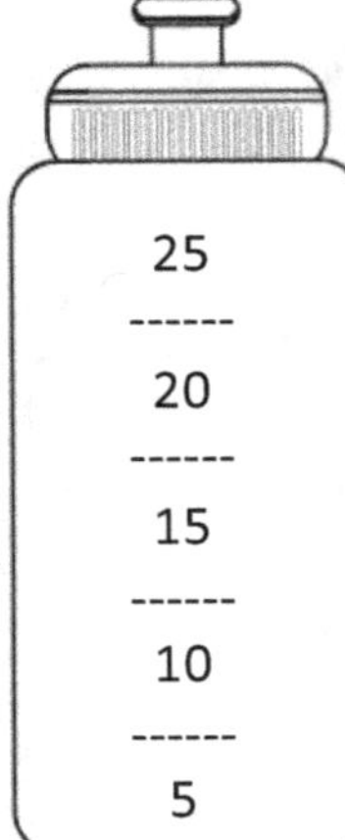

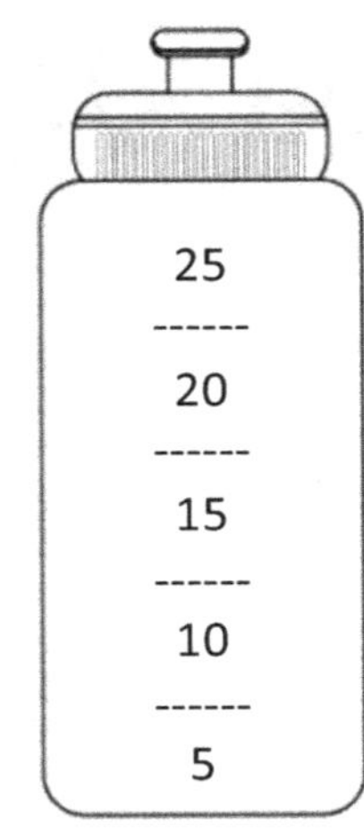

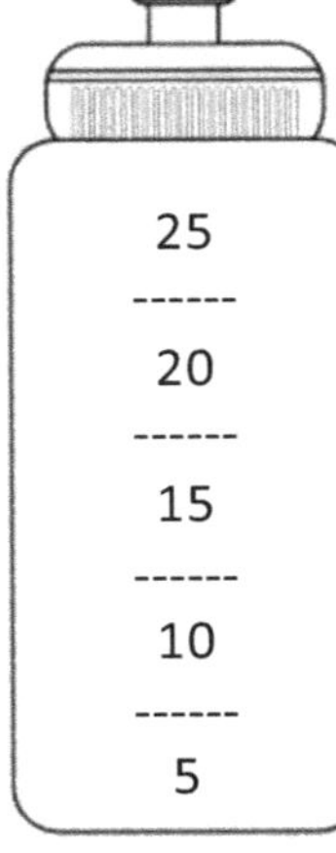

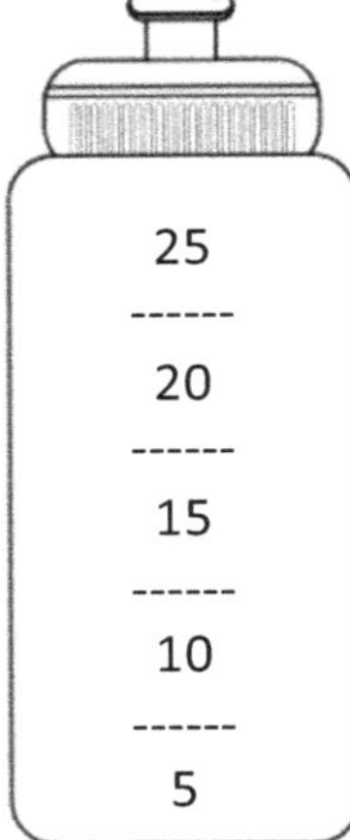

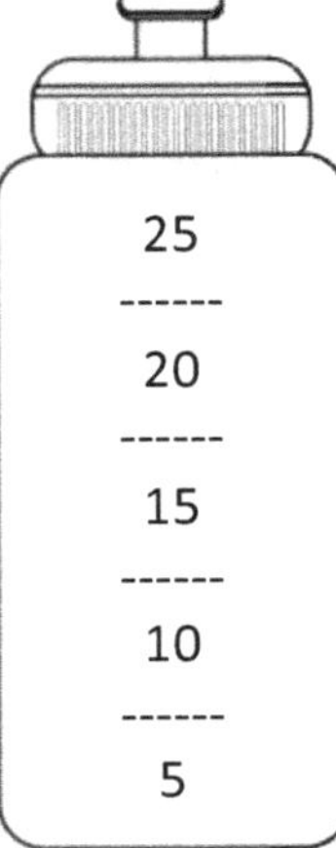

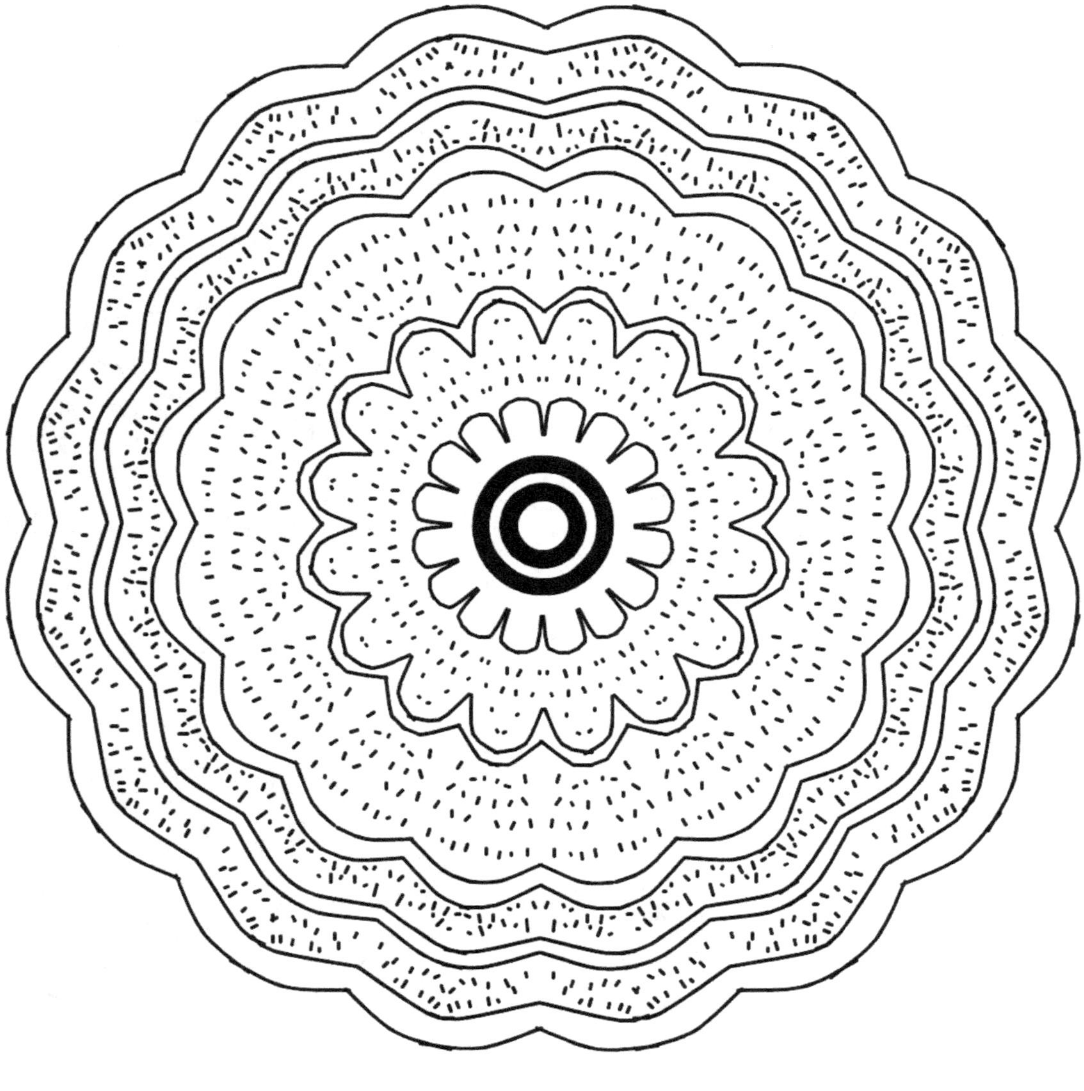

Day Eight _______

5:00 ____________________	

5:00 ______________________

6:00 ______________________

7:00 ______________________

8:00 ______________________

9:00 ______________________

10:00 ____________________

11:00 ____________________

Noon _____________________

1:00 ______________________

2:00 ______________________

3:00 ______________________

4:00 ______________________

5:00 ______________________

6:00 ______________________

7:00 ______________________

8:00 ______________________

9:00 ______________________

10:00 ____________________

11:00 ____________________

Midnight __________________

top priorities for today

____

____

____

____

Today's victories

What motivates you to be
the best version of you?

____

____

____

____

____

The Training

Exercise	Set 1	Set 2	Set 3	Set 4	Set 5	notes

Time started: _______________ Time ended: _______________

Location: ____

Feelings before training:

Feelings after training

NUTRITION

Meal 1
time eaten: _________

Meal 2
time eaten: _________

Meal 3
time eaten: _________

Meal 4
time eaten: _________

Meal 5
time eaten: _________

Hydration

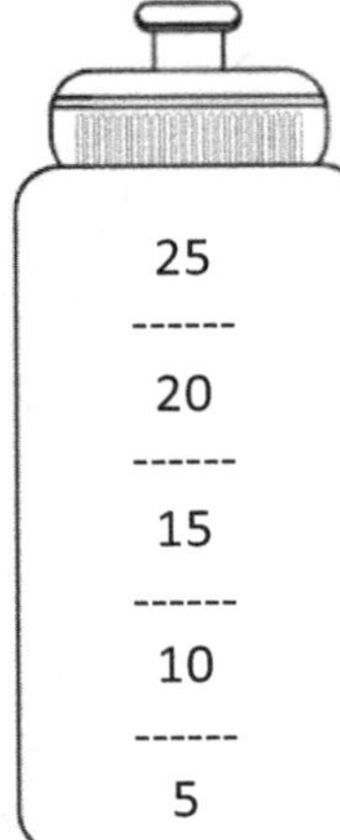

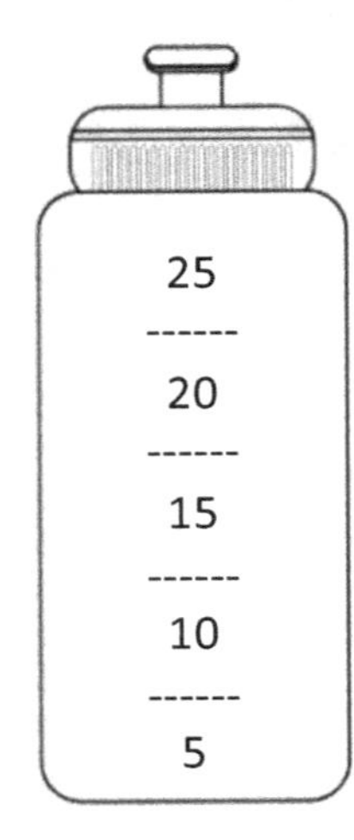

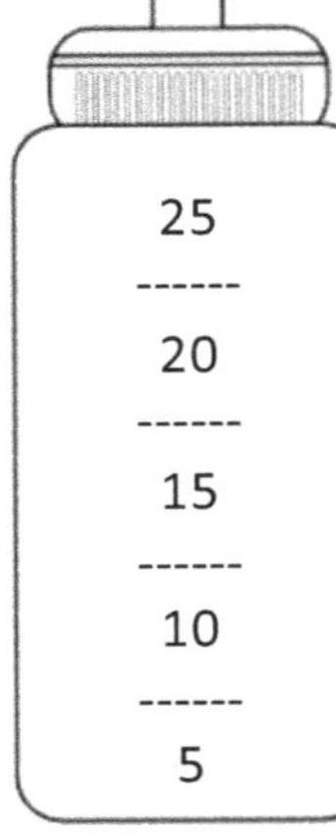

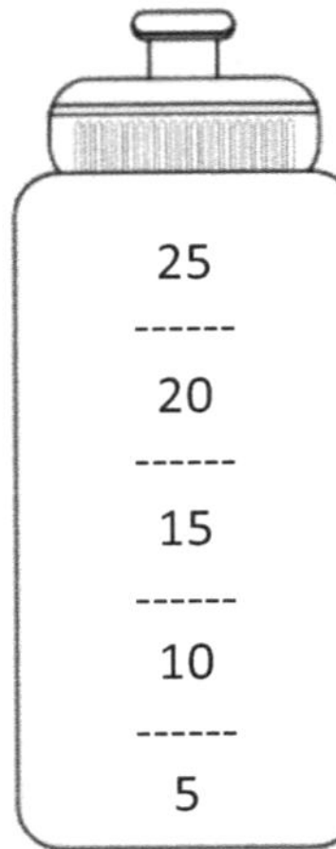

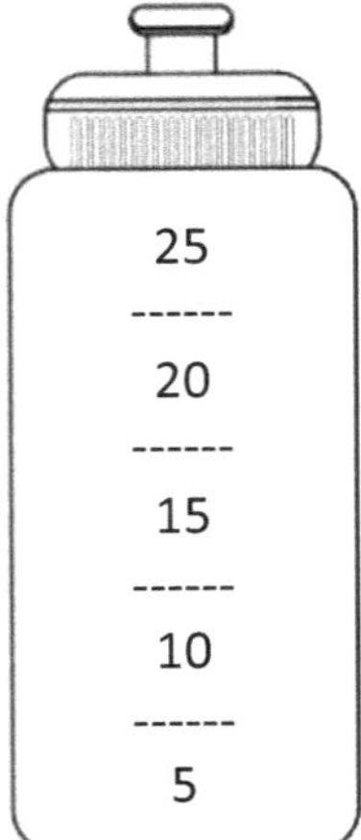

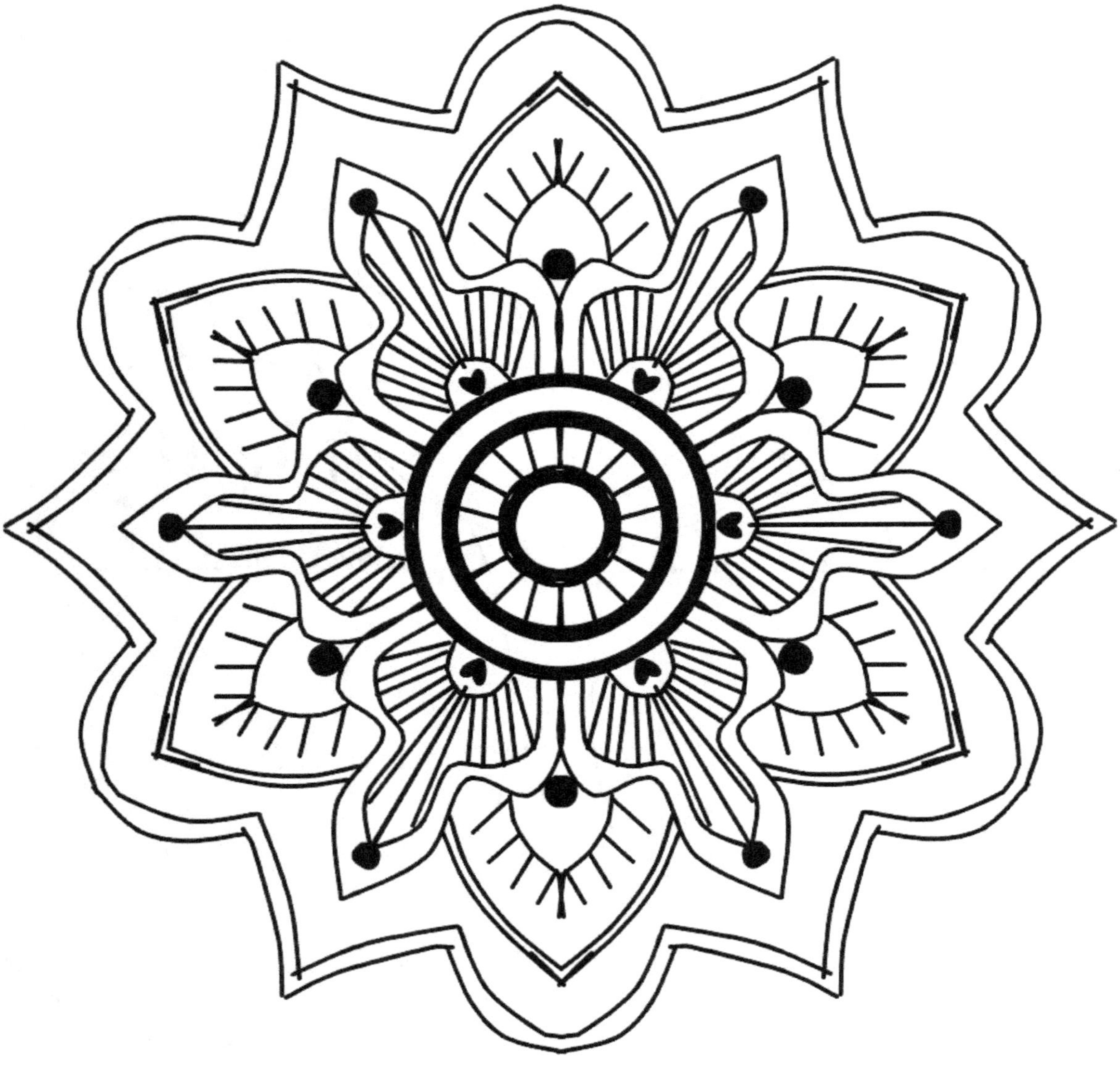

Day Nine _______

Time	
5:00	_________________
6:00	_________________
7:00	_________________
8:00	_________________
9:00	_________________
10:00	_________________
11:00	_________________
Noon	_________________
1:00	_________________
2:00	_________________
3:00	_________________
4:00	_________________
5:00	_________________
6:00	_________________
7:00	_________________
8:00	_________________
9:00	_________________
10:00	_________________
11:00	_________________
Midnight	_________________

top priorities for today

____
____
____
____
____

Today's victories

How will you be consistent this week?

____
____
____
____
____
____

The Stella Society Training

Exercise	Set 1	Set 2	Set 3	Set 4	Set 5	notes

Time started: _____________ Time ended: _______________

Location: ____

Feelings before training: 🙂 😐 🙁 😜 😠 😟 😊 😎

Feelings after training 🙂 😐 🙁 😜 😠 😟 😊 😎

NUTRITION

Meal 1
time eaten: _________

Meal 2
time eaten: _________

Meal 3
time eaten: _________

Meal 4
time eaten: _________

Meal 5
time eaten: _________

Hydration

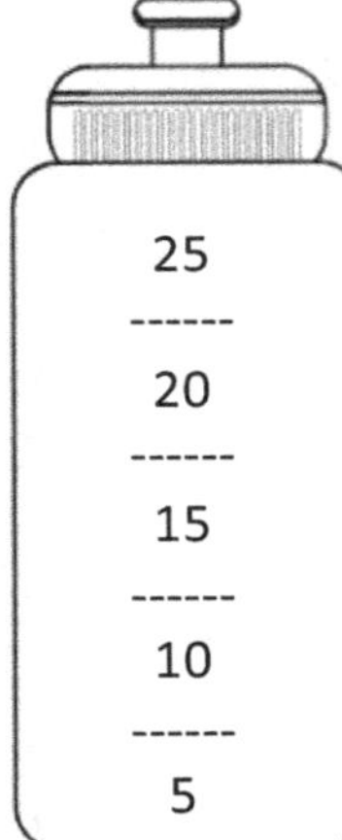

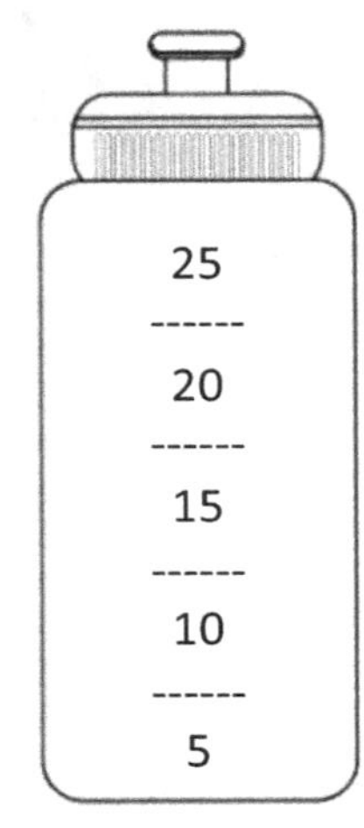

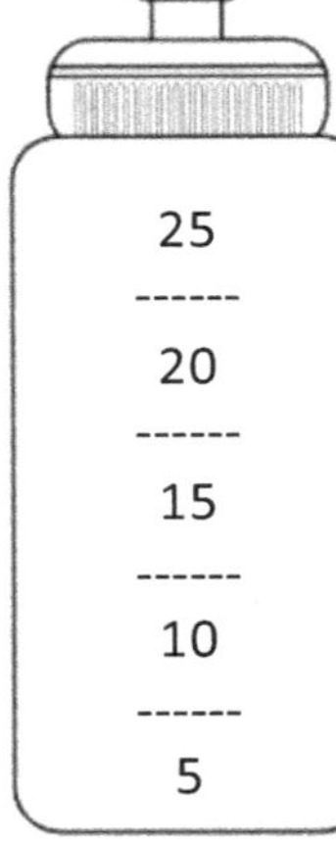

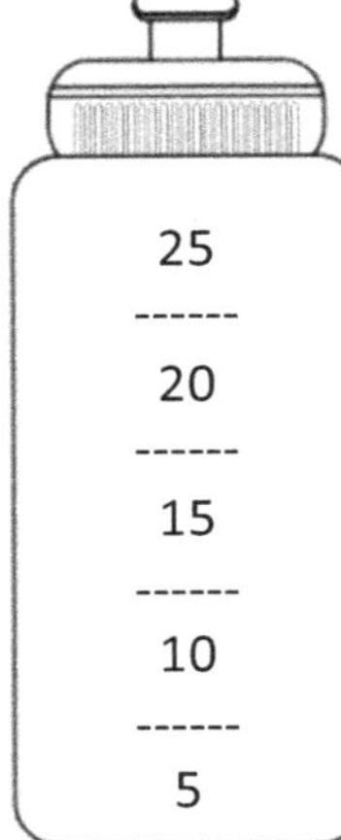

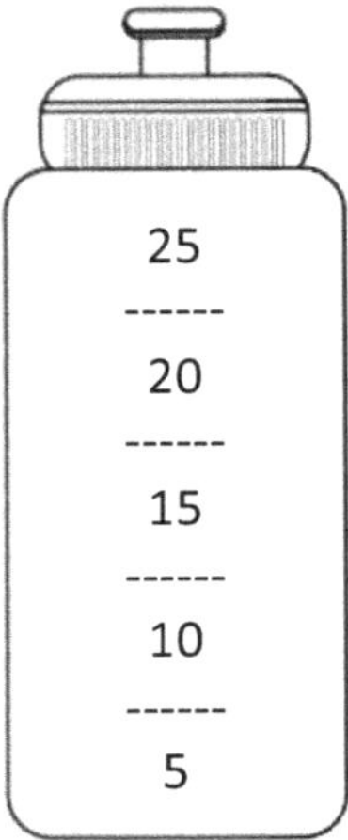

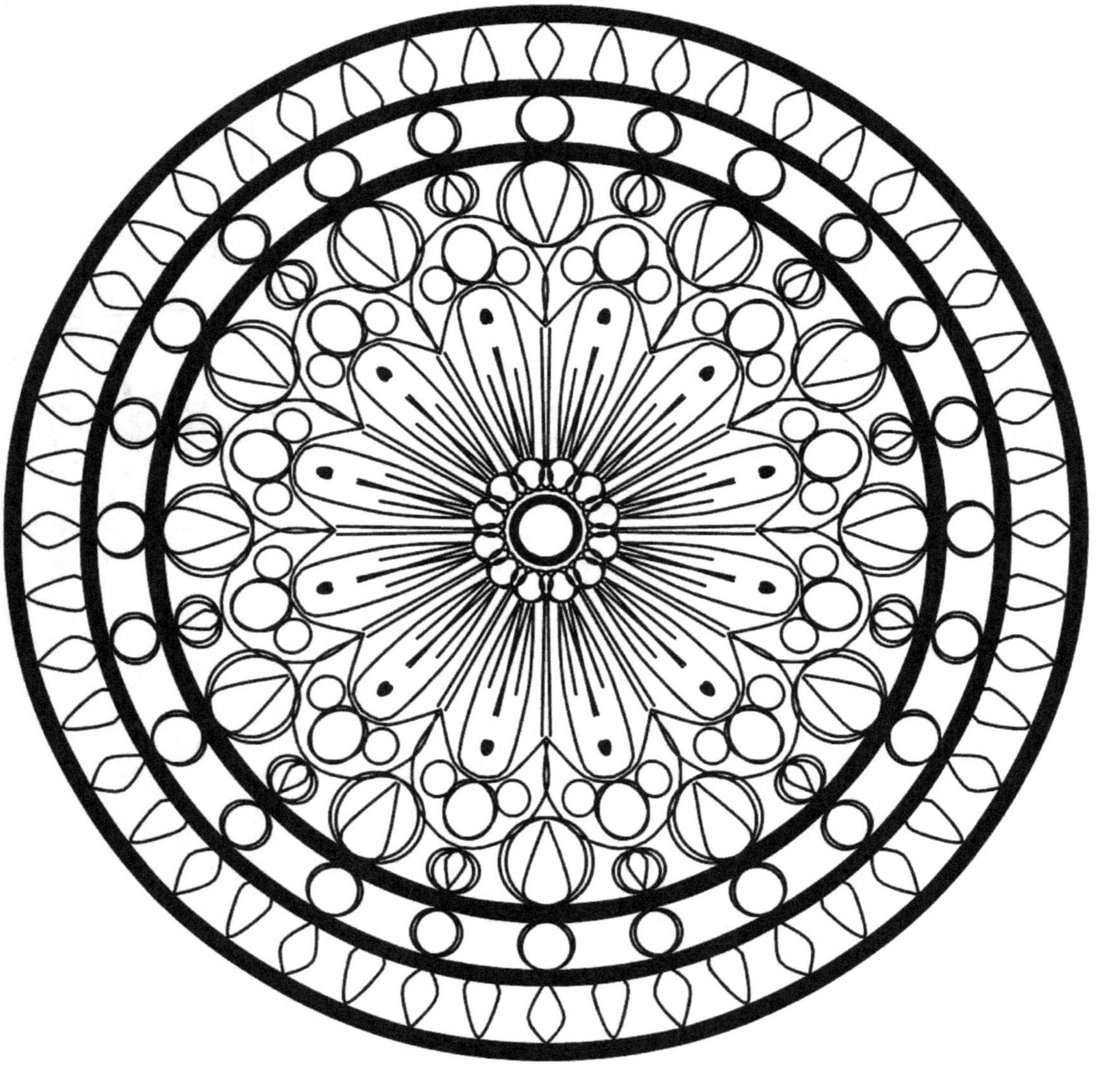

Day Ten _______

5:00 _______________________

6:00 _______________________

7:00 _______________________

8:00 _______________________

9:00 _______________________

10:00 _______________________

11:00 _______________________

Noon _______________________

1:00 _______________________

2:00 _______________________

3:00 _______________________

4:00 _______________________

5:00 _______________________

6:00 _______________________

7:00 _______________________

8:00 _______________________

9:00 _______________________

10:00 _______________________

11:00 _______________________

Midnight _______________________

top priorities for today

____

____

____

____

Today's victories

List 5 ways you are loving.

____

____

____

____

____

The Stella Society Training

Exercise	Set 1	Set 2	Set 3	Set 4	Set 5	notes

Time started: _____________ Time ended: _____________

Location: ____

Feelings before training: 😊 😐 ☹️ 😜 😣 😟 😇 😎

Feelings after training 😊 😐 ☹️ 😜 😣 😟 😇 😎

NUTRITION

Meal 1
time eaten: _________

Meal 2
time eaten: _________

Meal 3
time eaten: _________

Meal 4
time eaten: _________

Meal 5
time eaten: _________

Hydration

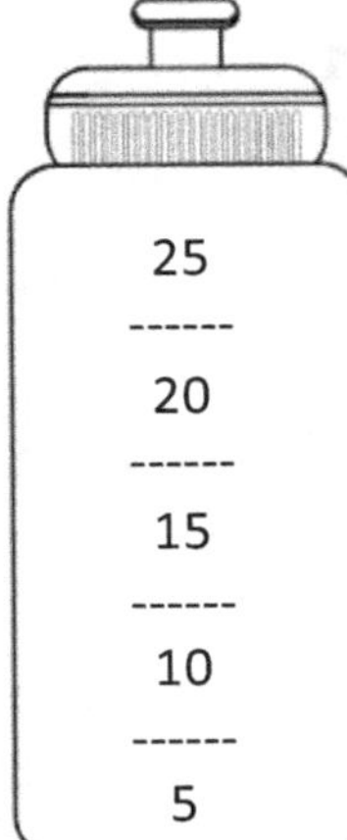
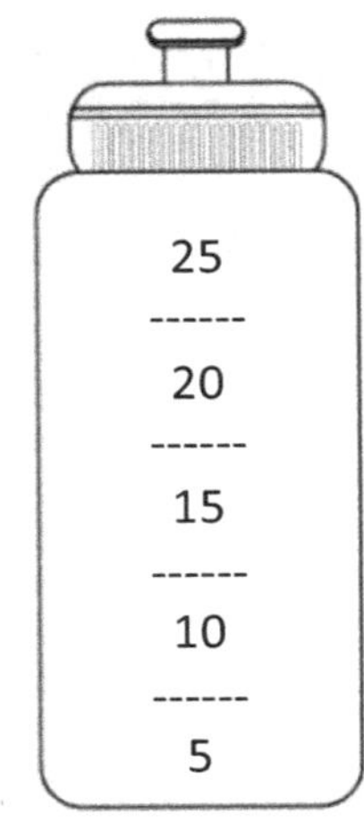
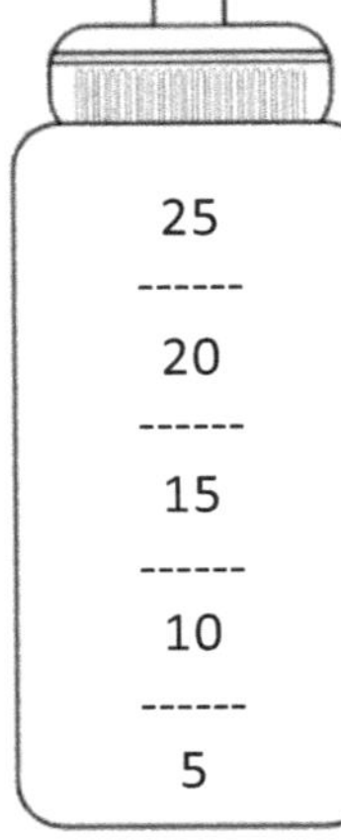
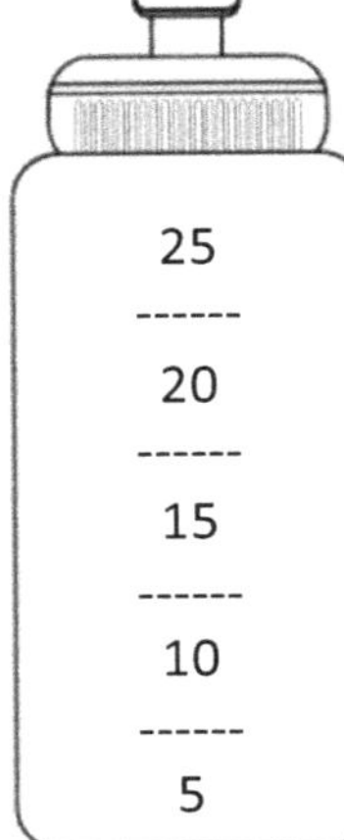
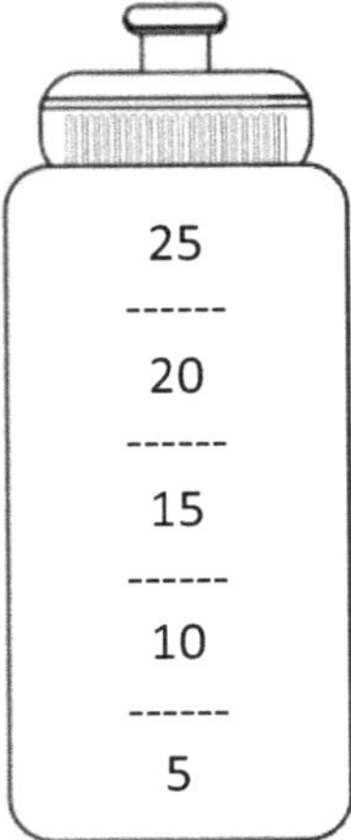

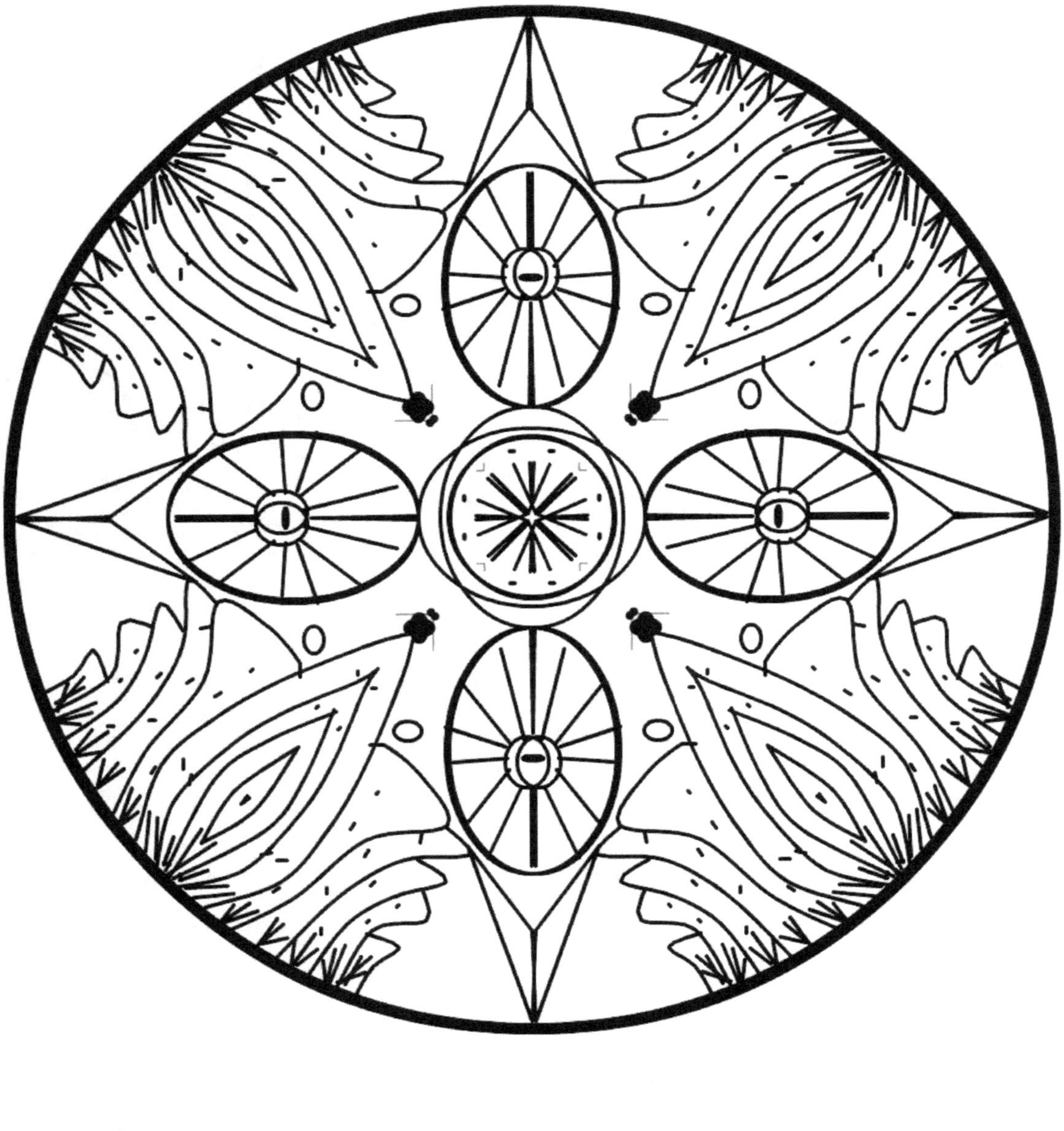

Measurements

P R O G R E S S

DATE: _____________

Weight: _______

Neck _______

Shoulders _______

Chest _______

Bicep / upper arm left _________ right ________

Forearm left _________ right ________

Waist _______

Hips _______

Thighs left _________ right _____

Calf left _________ right ________

C H E C K

The Struggle You Are In Today, Is Developing The Strength You Need for Tomorrow.

5:00 ________________________

6:00 ________________________

7:00 ________________________

8:00 ________________________

9:00 ________________________

10:00 ________________________

11:00 ________________________

Noon ________________________

1:00 ________________________

2:00 ________________________

3:00 ________________________

4:00 ________________________

5:00 ________________________

6:00 ________________________

7:00 ________________________

8:00 ________________________

9:00 ________________________

10:00 ________________________

11:00 ________________________

Midnight ________________________

____

____

____

____

____

Give out as many hugs as you can today. How many did you give?

____

____

____

____

____

____

The Training

Exercise	Set 1	Set 2	Set 3	Set 4	Set 5	notes

Time started: _____________ Time ended: _____________

Location: ____

Feelings before training: 🙂 😐 🙁 😜 😠 😟 😊 😎

Feelings after training 🙂 😐 🙁 😜 😠 😟 😊 😎

NUTRITION

Meal 1
time eaten: _________

Meal 2
time eaten: _________

Meal 3
time eaten: _________

Meal 4
time eaten: _________

Meal 5
time eaten: _________

Hydration

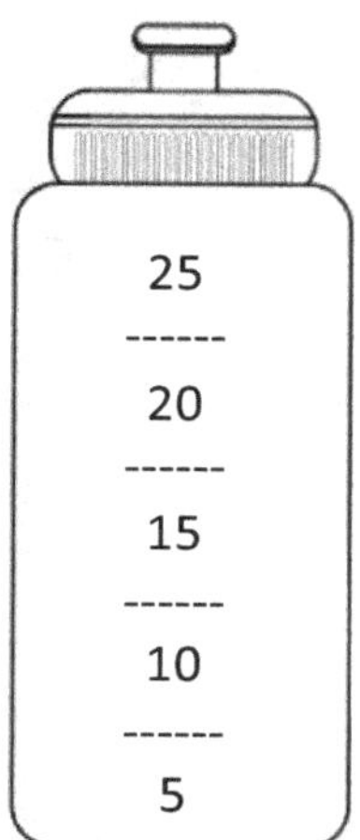

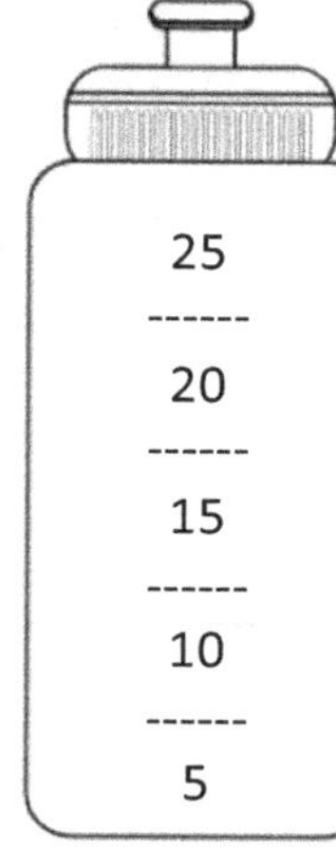

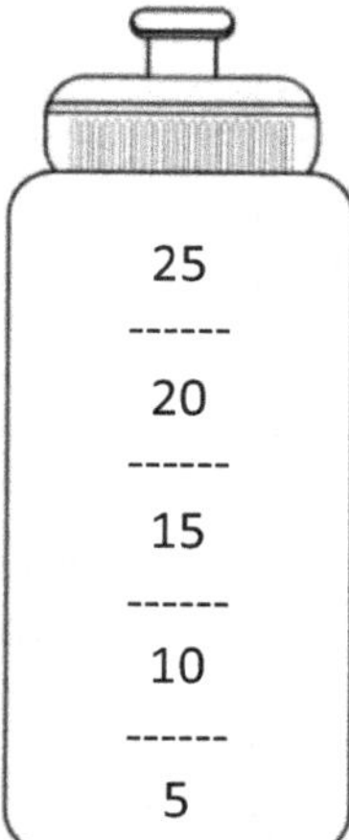

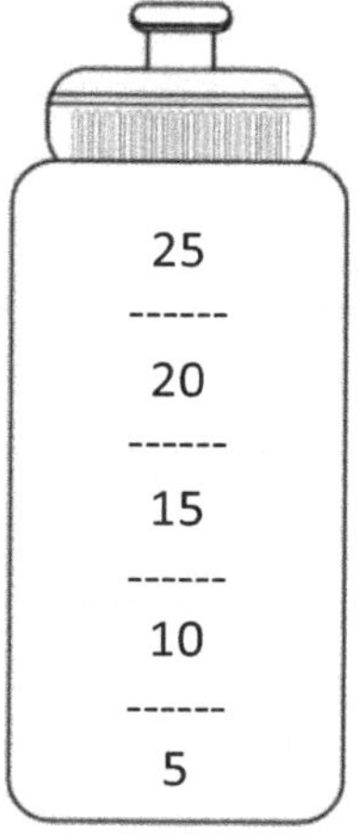

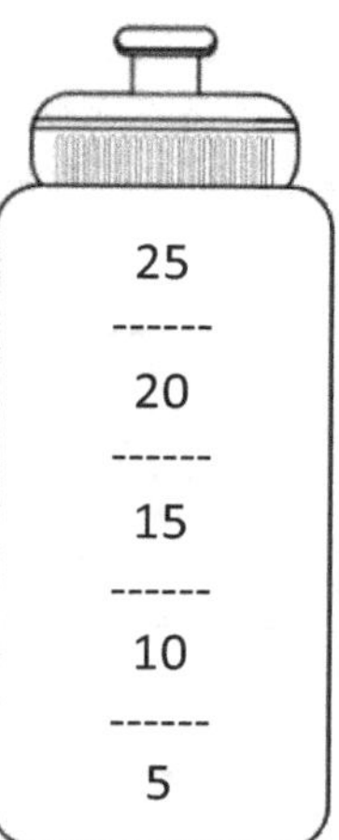

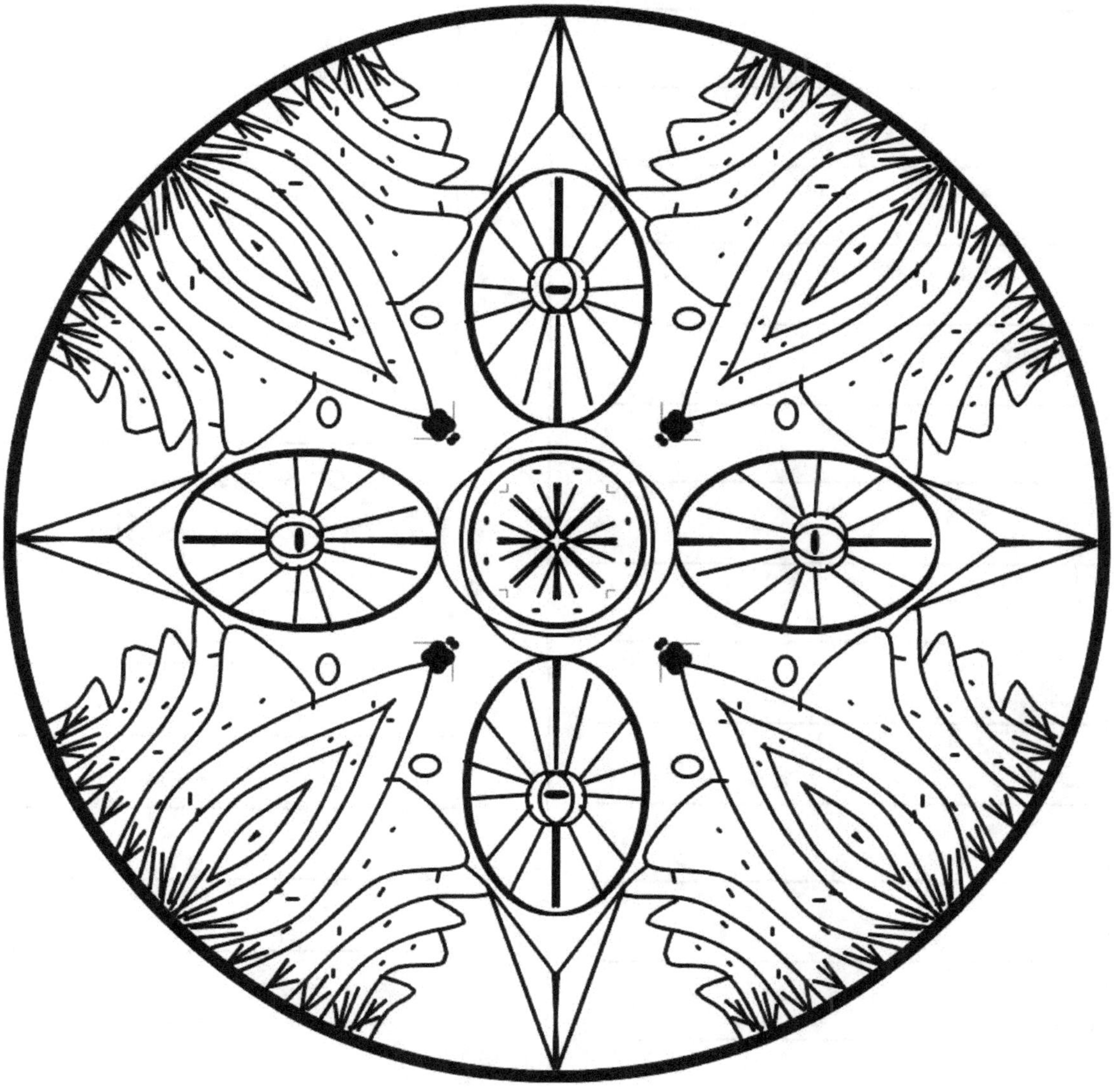

Day Twelve _______

5:00 _______________________

6:00 _______________________

7:00 _______________________

8:00 _______________________

9:00 _______________________

10:00 ______________________

11:00 ______________________

Noon _______________________

1:00 _______________________

2:00 _______________________

3:00 _______________________

4:00 _______________________

5:00 _______________________

6:00 _______________________

7:00 _______________________

8:00 _______________________

9:00 _______________________

10:00 ______________________

11:00 ______________________

Midnight ____________________

Today's victories

List 4 ways you show compassion.

The Stella Society Training

Exercise	Set 1	Set 2	Set 3	Set 4	Set 5	notes

Time started: _____________ Time ended: _____________

Location: ____

Feelings before training:

Feelings after training

NUTRITION

Meal 1
time eaten: _________

Meal 2
time eaten: _________

Meal 3
time eaten: _________

Meal 4
time eaten: _________

Meal 5
time eaten: _________

Hydration

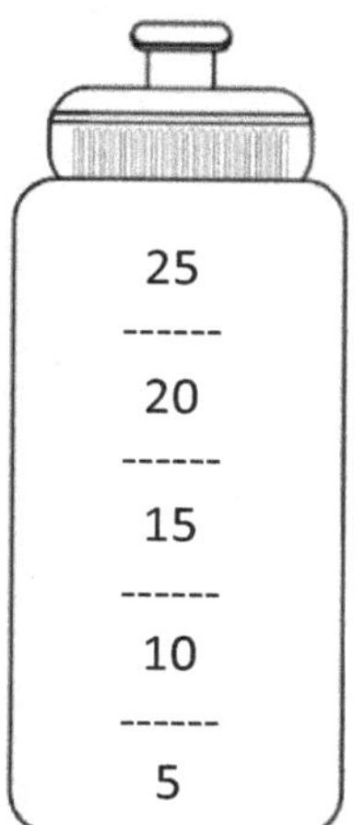

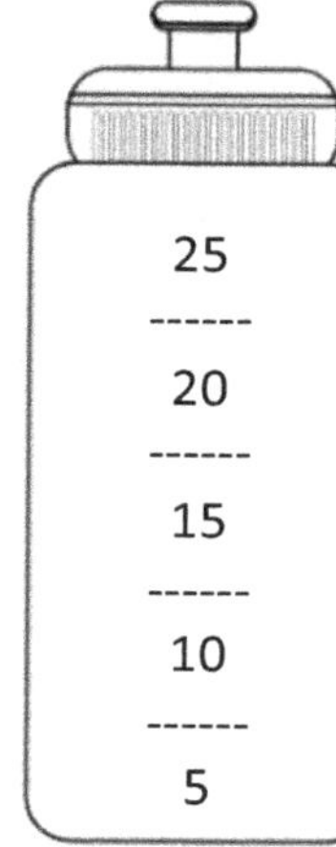

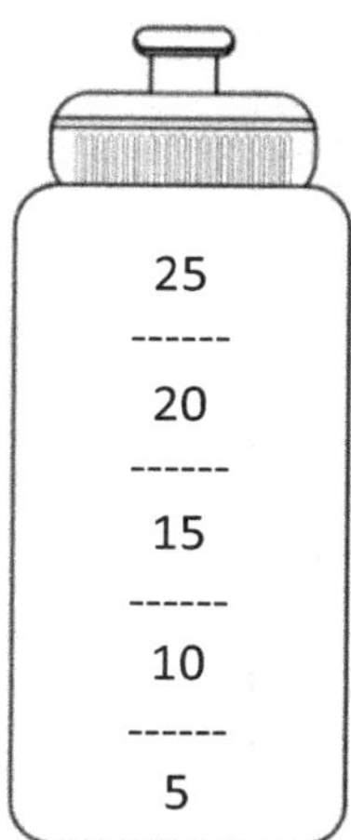

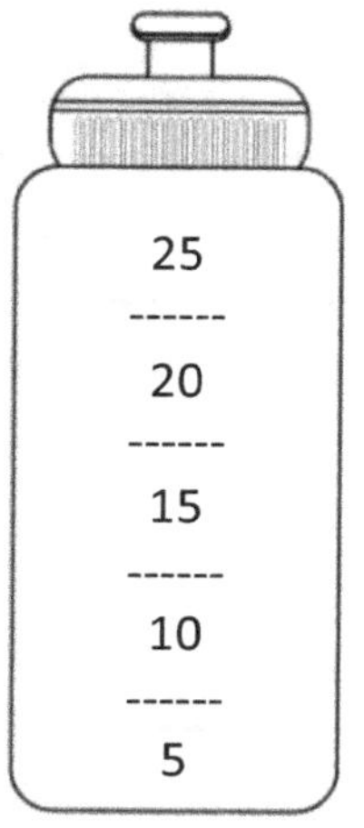

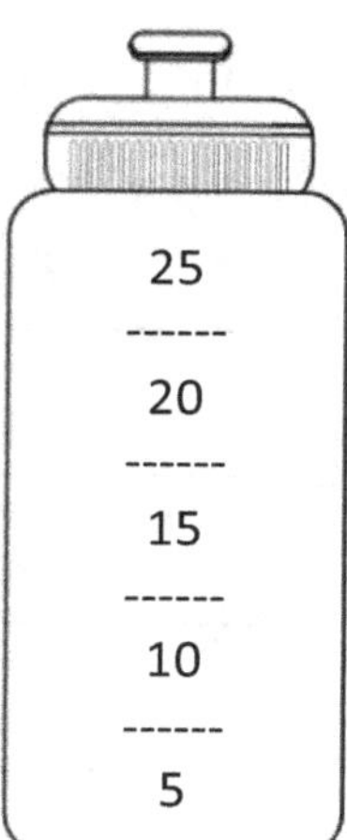

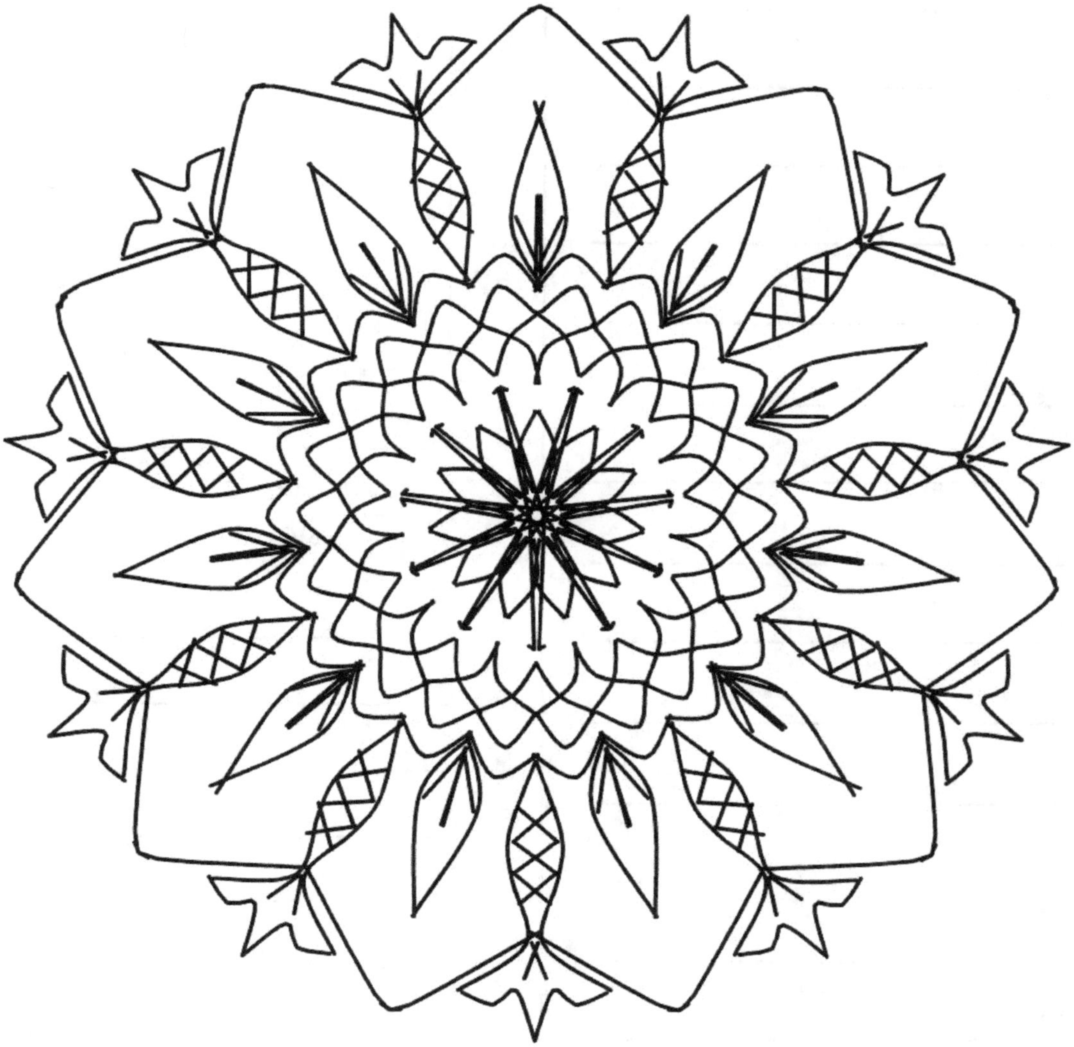

Day Thirteen _______

5:00 _______________________

6:00 _______________________

7:00 _______________________

8:00 _______________________

9:00 _______________________

10:00 _______________________

11:00 _______________________

Noon _______________________

1:00 _______________________

2:00 _______________________

3:00 _______________________

4:00 _______________________

5:00 _______________________

6:00 _______________________

7:00 _______________________

8:00 _______________________

9:00 _______________________

10:00 _______________________

11:00 _______________________

Midnight _______________________

top priorities for today

____

____

____

____

____

Today's victories

Who needs roses from your garden and why?

____

____

____

____

____

____

The Training

Exercise	Set 1	Set 2	Set 3	Set 4	Set 5	notes

Time started: _____________ Time ended: _____________

Location: ____

Feelings before training:

Feelings after training

NUTRITION

Meal 1
time eaten: _________

Meal 2
time eaten: _________

Meal 3
time eaten: _________

Meal 4
time eaten: _________

Meal 5
time eaten: _________

Hydration

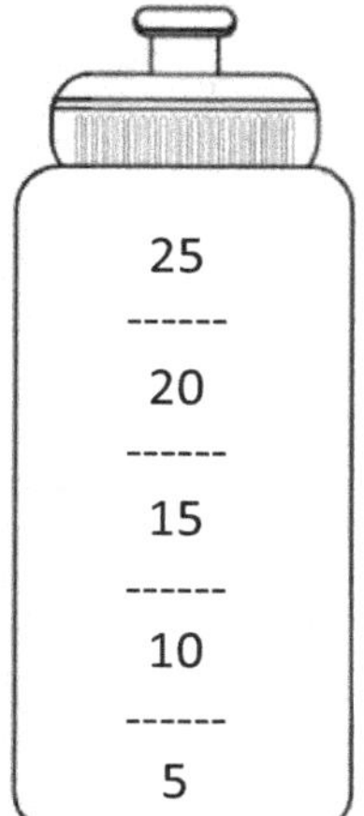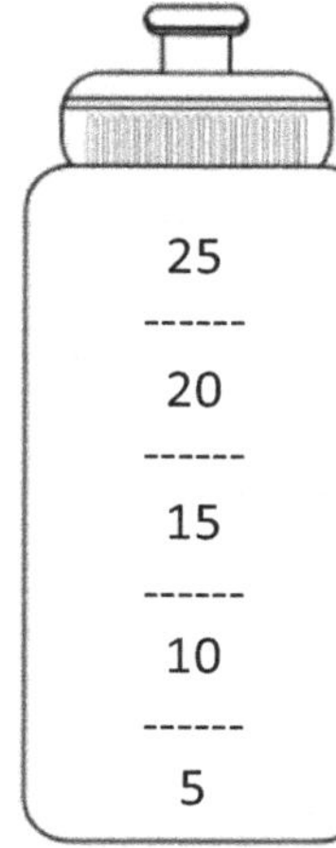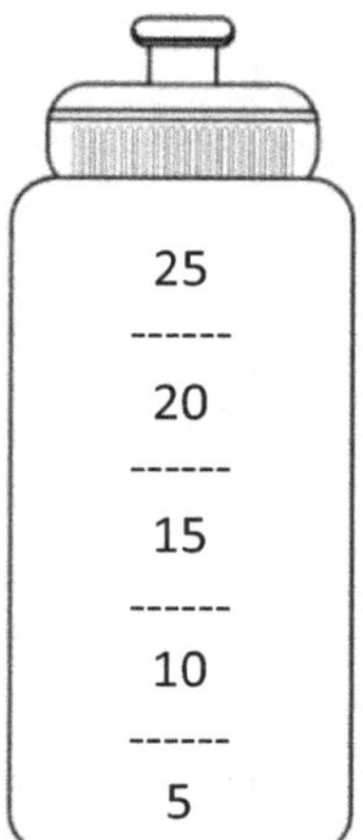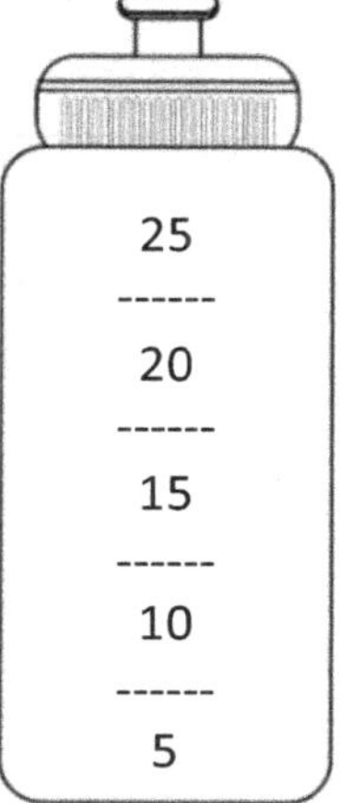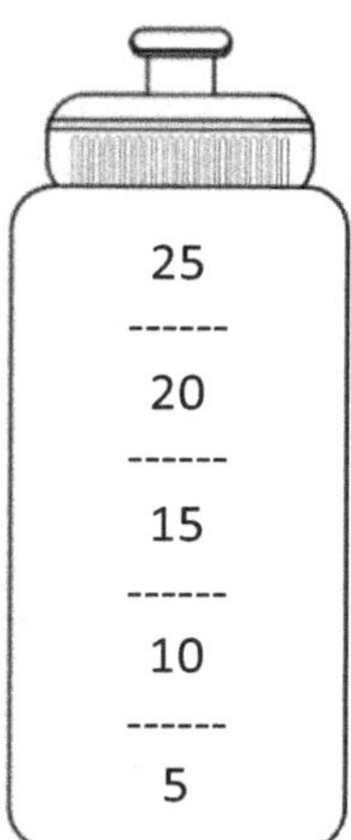

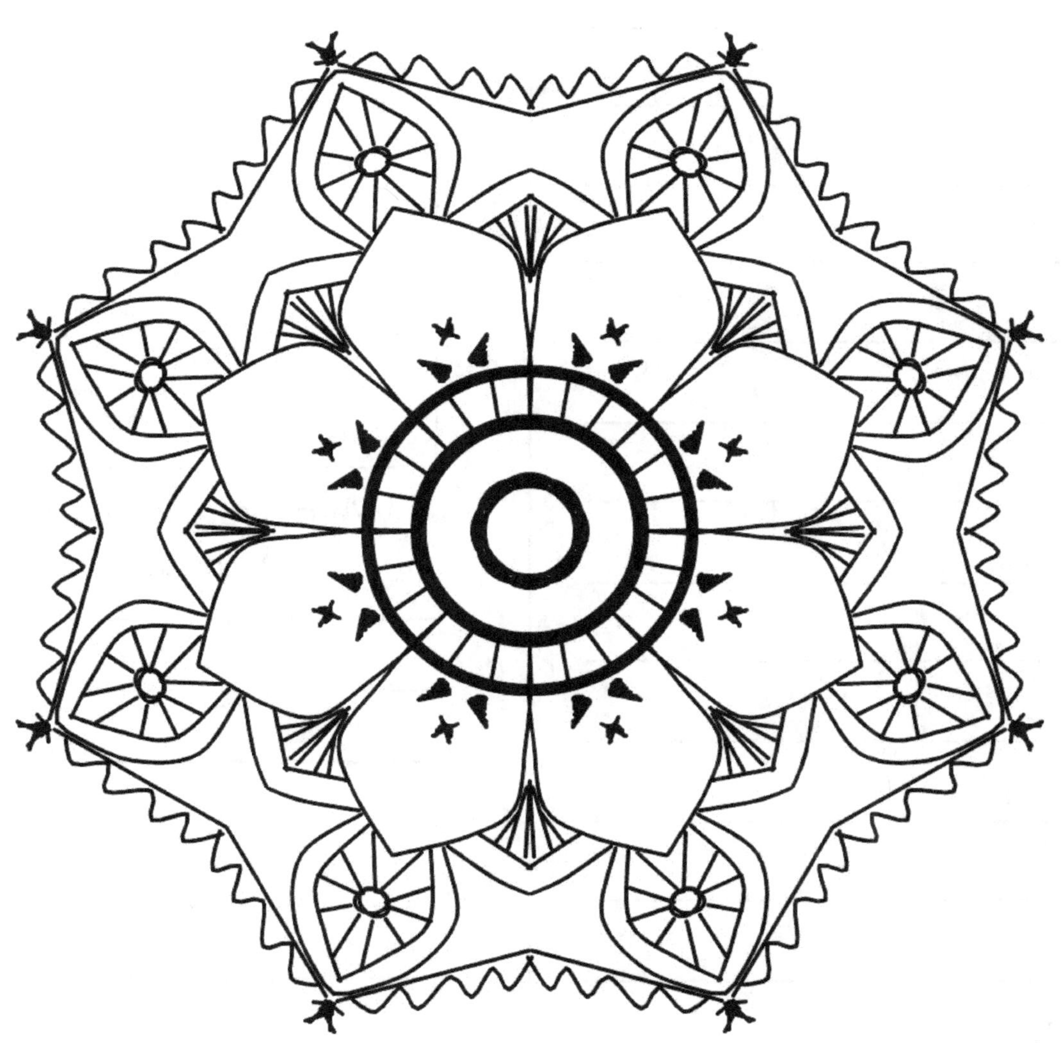

Day Fourteen ________

5:00 _______________________

6:00 _______________________

7:00 _______________________

8:00 _______________________

9:00 _______________________

10:00 ______________________

11:00 ______________________

Noon _______________________

1:00 _______________________

2:00 _______________________

3:00 _______________________

4:00 _______________________

5:00 _______________________

6:00 _______________________

7:00 _______________________

8:00 _______________________

9:00 _______________________

10:00 ______________________

11:00 ______________________

Midnight ___________________

top priorities for today 🎯

____

____

____

____

____

Today's victories 🏆

What should you forgive
your self for?

____

____

____

____

____

The Training

Exercise	Set 1	Set 2	Set 3	Set 4	Set 5	notes

Time started: _______________ Time ended: _______________

Location: ____

Feelings before training:

Feelings after training

NUTRITION

Meal 1

time eaten: _________

Meal 2

time eaten: _________

Meal 3

time eaten: _________

Meal 4

time eaten: _________

Meal 5

time eaten: _________

Hydration

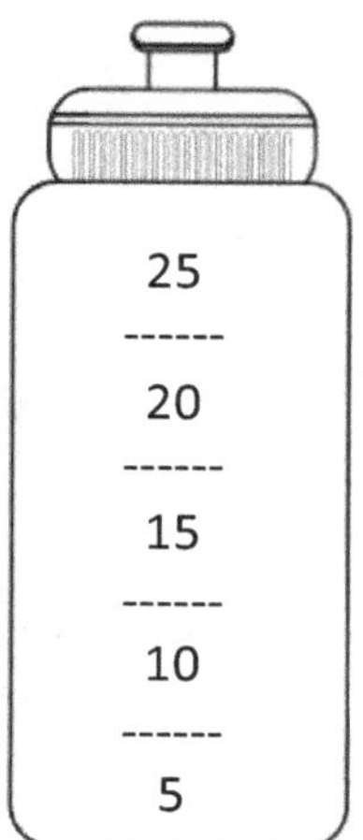
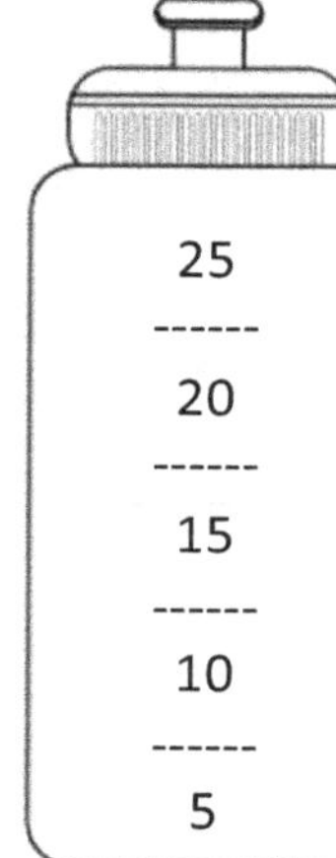
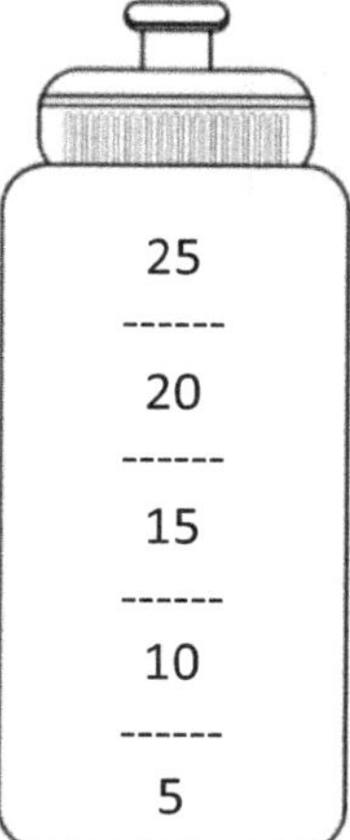
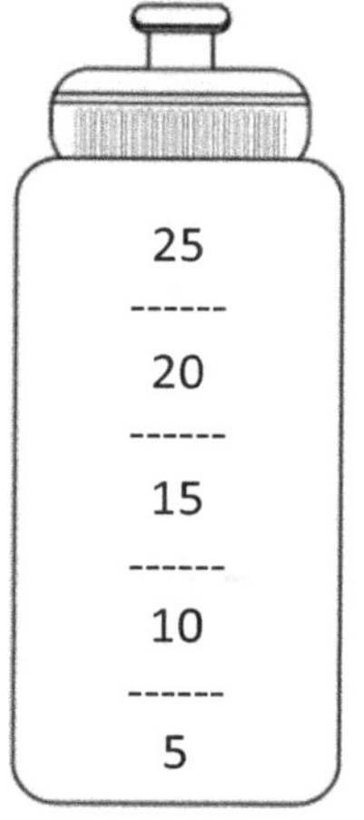
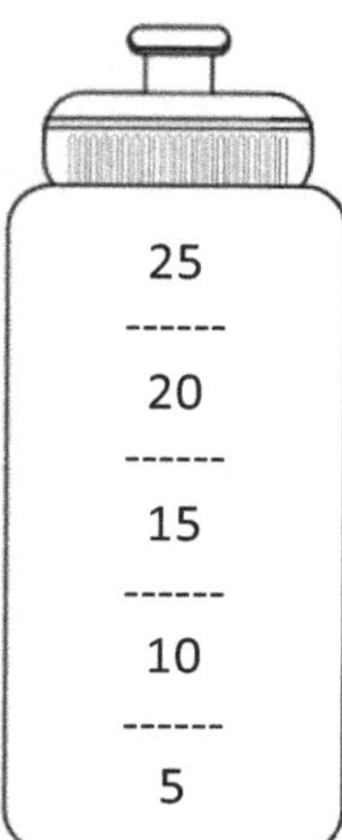

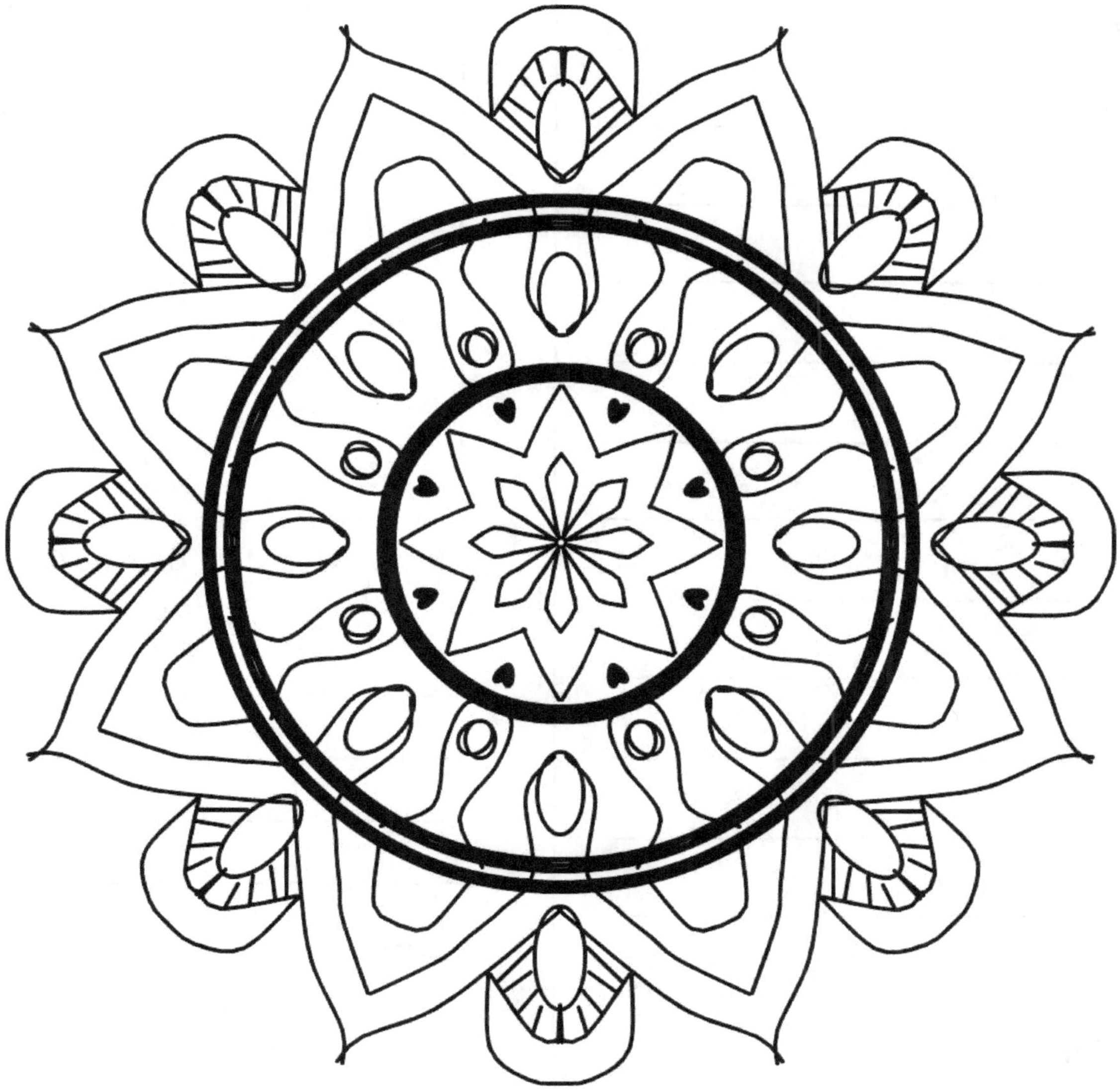

Day Fifteen _______

5:00 _______________________

6:00 _______________________

7:00 _______________________

8:00 _______________________

9:00 _______________________

10:00 ______________________

11:00 ______________________

Noon _______________________

1:00 _______________________

2:00 _______________________

3:00 _______________________

4:00 _______________________

5:00 _______________________

6:00 _______________________

7:00 _______________________

8:00 _______________________

9:00 _______________________

10:00 ______________________

11:00 ______________________

Midnight ___________________

top priorities for today

____

____

____

____

Today's victories

How will you be remarkable today?

____

____

____

____

____

____

The Training

Exercise	Set 1	Set 2	Set 3	Set 4	Set 5	notes

Time started: ______________ Time ended: ______________

Location: ____

Feelings before training:

Feelings after training

NUTRITION

Meal 1
time eaten: _________

Meal 2
time eaten: _________

Meal 3
time eaten: _________

Meal 4
time eaten: _________

Meal 5
time eaten: _________

Hydration

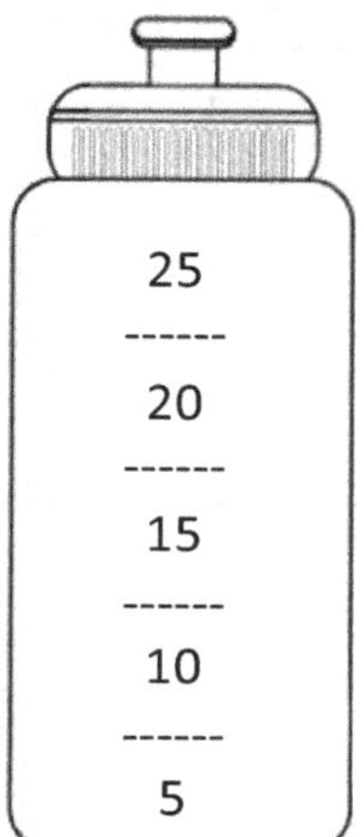

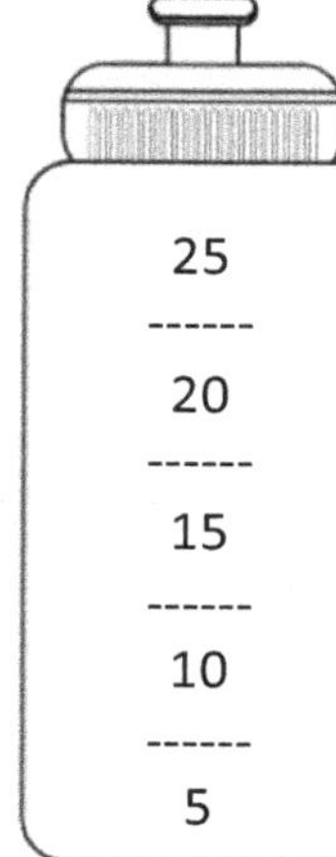

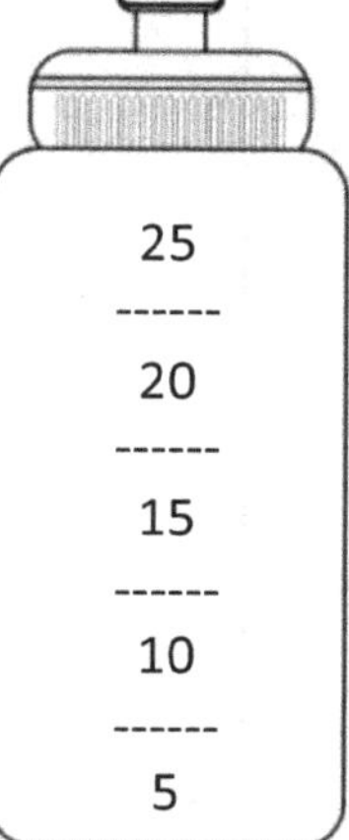

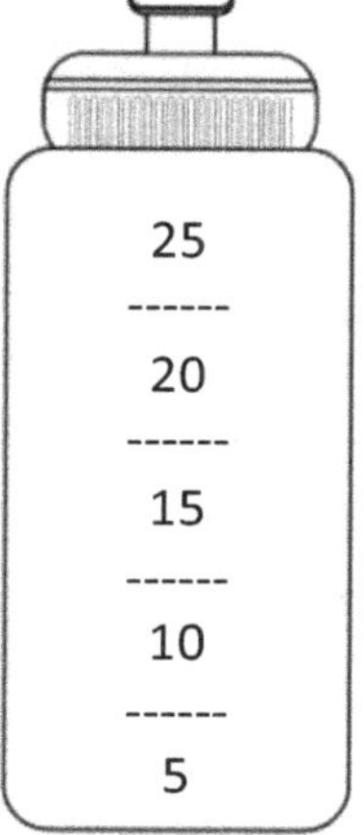

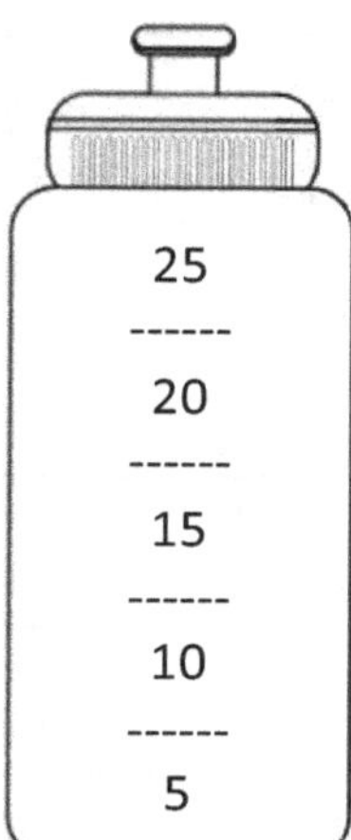

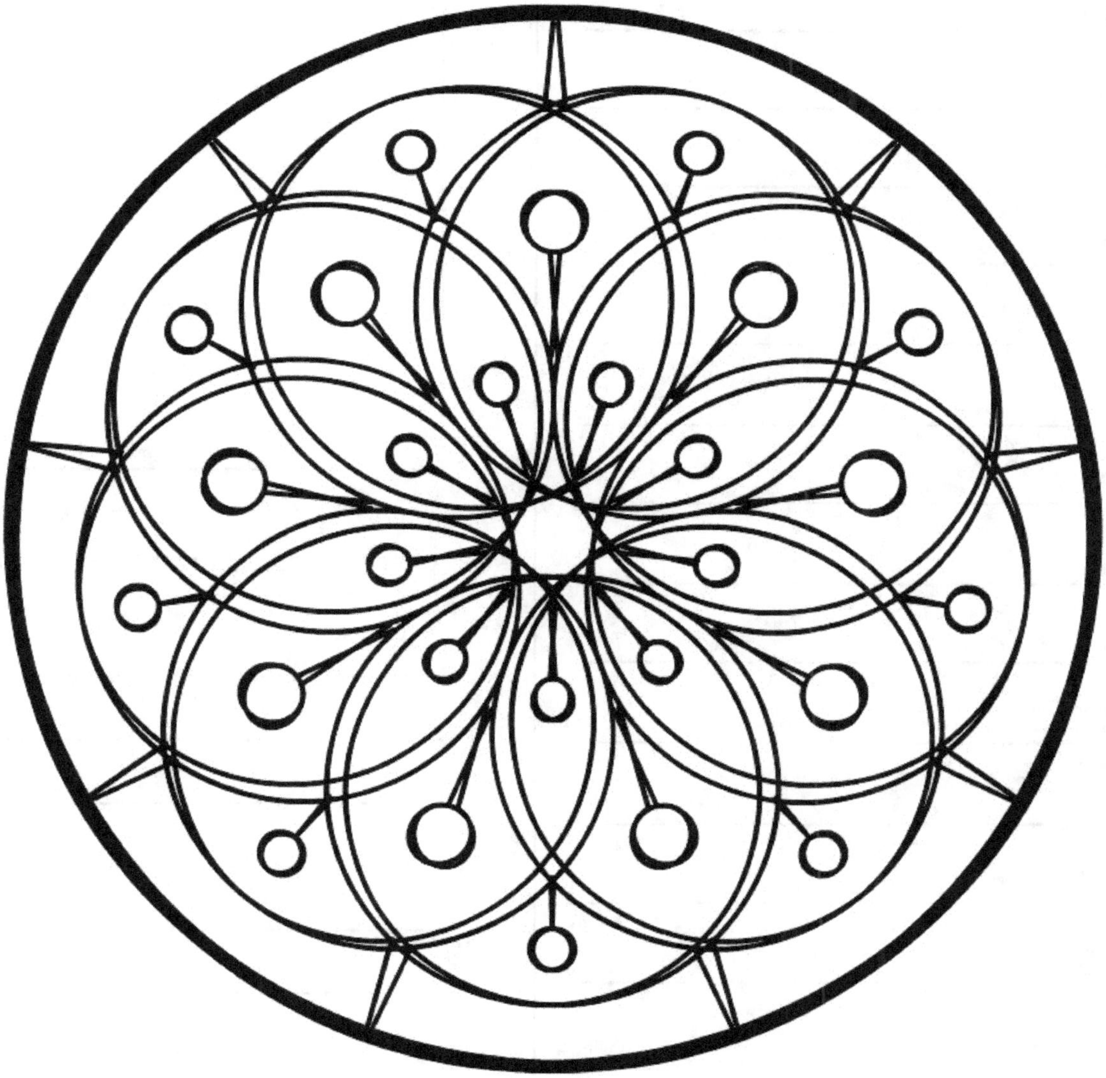

Day Sixteen _______

5:00 _______________________

6:00 _______________________

7:00 _______________________

8:00 _______________________

9:00 _______________________

10:00 ______________________

11:00 ______________________

Noon _______________________

1:00 _______________________

2:00 _______________________

3:00 _______________________

4:00 _______________________

5:00 _______________________

6:00 _______________________

7:00 _______________________

8:00 _______________________

9:00 _______________________

10:00 ______________________

11:00 ______________________

Midnight ___________________

____

____

____

____

____

Watch the sunset and list 5 places you want to see it happen?

____

____

____

____

____

____

The Training

Exercise	Set 1	Set 2	Set 3	Set 4	Set 5	notes

Time started: _____________ Time ended: _____________

Location: ____

Feelings before training:

Feelings after training

NUTRITION

Meal 1

time eaten: _________

Meal 2

time eaten: _________

Meal 3

time eaten: _________

Meal 4

time eaten: _________

Meal 5

time eaten: _________

Hydration

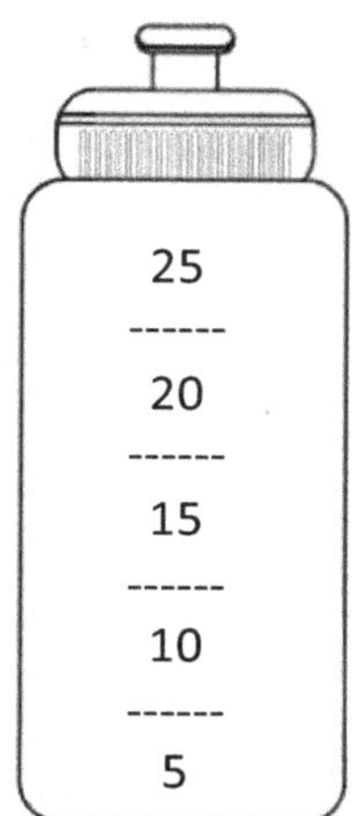
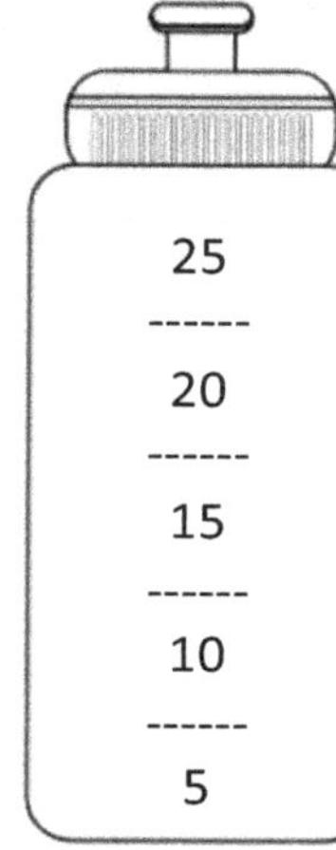
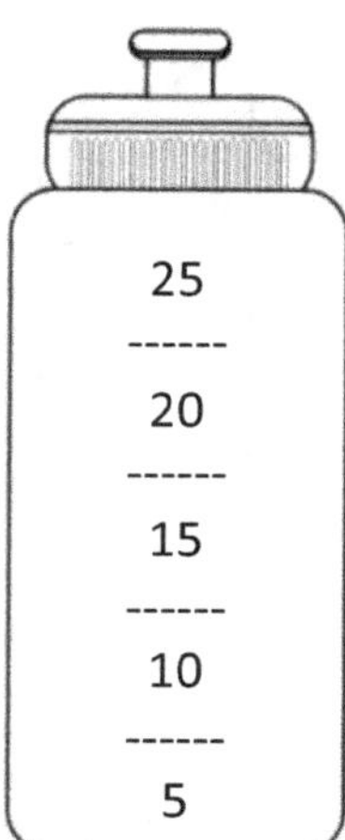
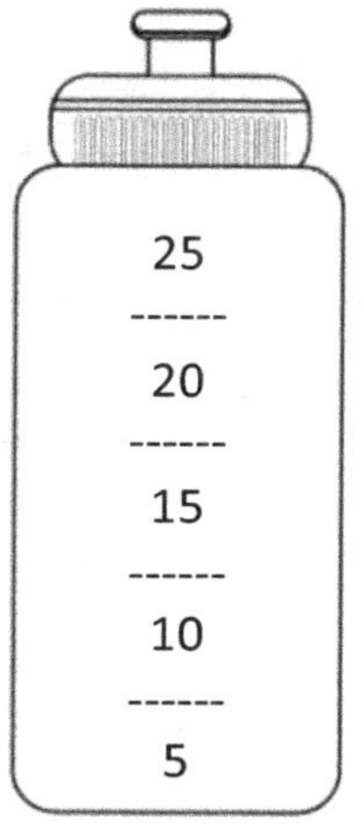
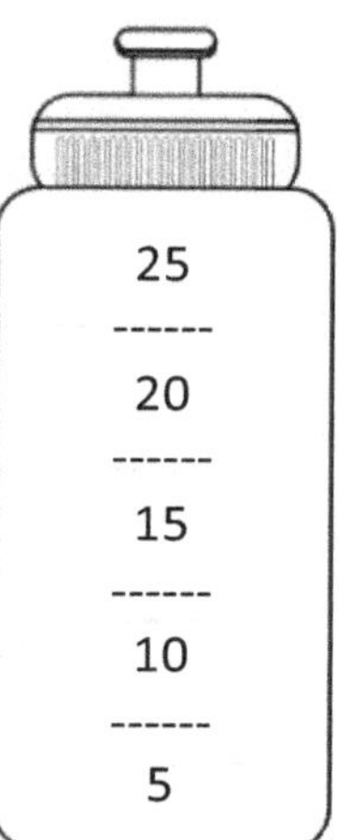

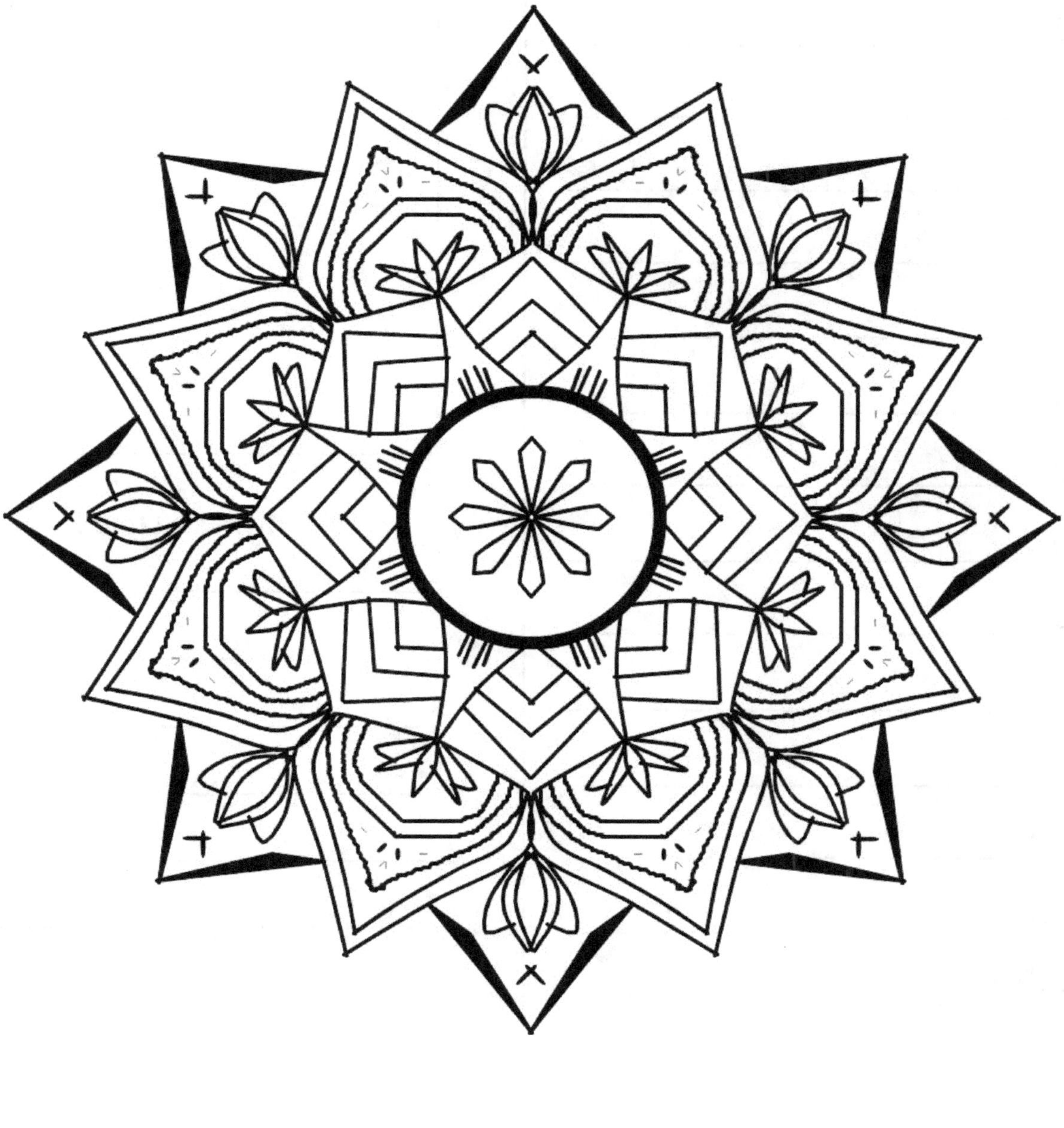

Day Seventeen _______

5:00 ______________

6:00 ______________

7:00 ______________

8:00 ______________

9:00 ______________

10:00 ______________

11:00 ______________

Noon ______________

1:00 ______________

2:00 ______________

3:00 ______________

4:00 ______________

5:00 ______________

6:00 ______________

7:00 ______________

8:00 ______________

9:00 ______________

10:00 ______________

11:00 ______________

Midnight ______________

top priorities for today

____

____

____

____

Today's victories

What makes you happy?

____

____

____

____

____

____

The Stella Society Training

Exercise	Set 1	Set 2	Set 3	Set 4	Set 5	notes

Time started: _____________ Time ended: _____________

Location: _______________________________________

Feelings before training:

Feelings after training

NUTRITION

Meal 1

time eaten: _________

Meal 2

time eaten: _________

Meal 3

time eaten: _________

Meal 4

time eaten: _________

Meal 5

time eaten: _________

Hydration

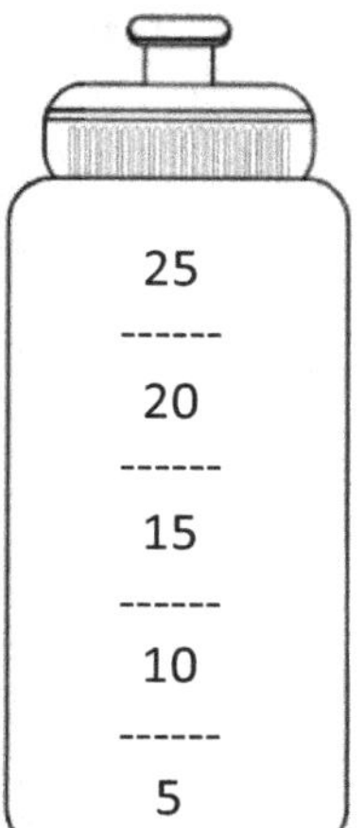
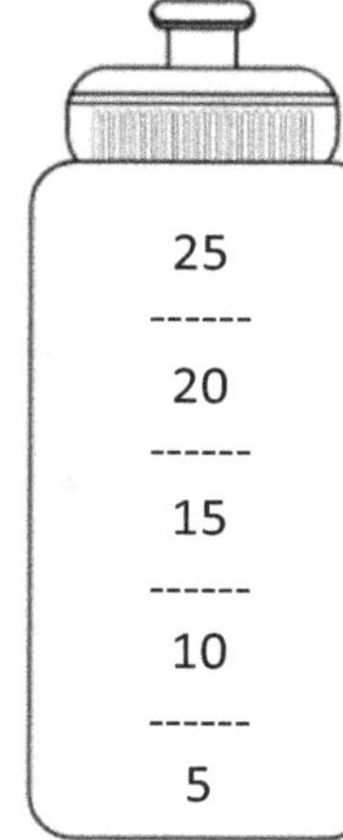
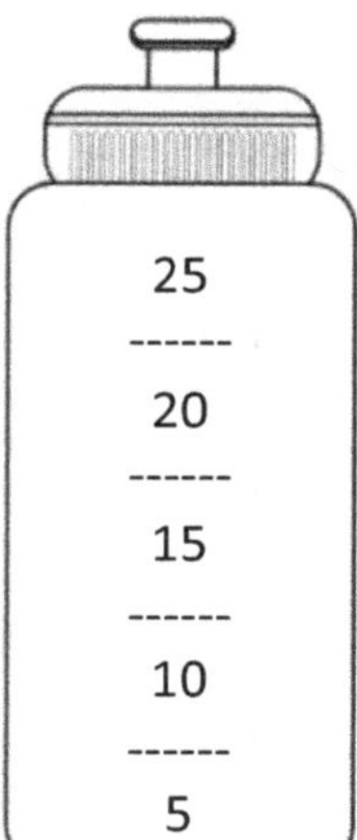
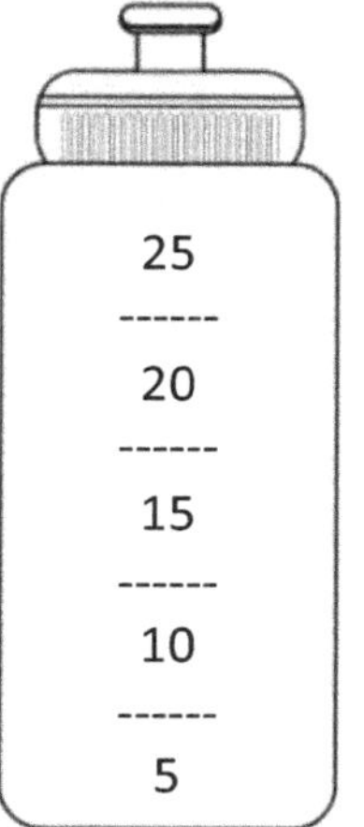
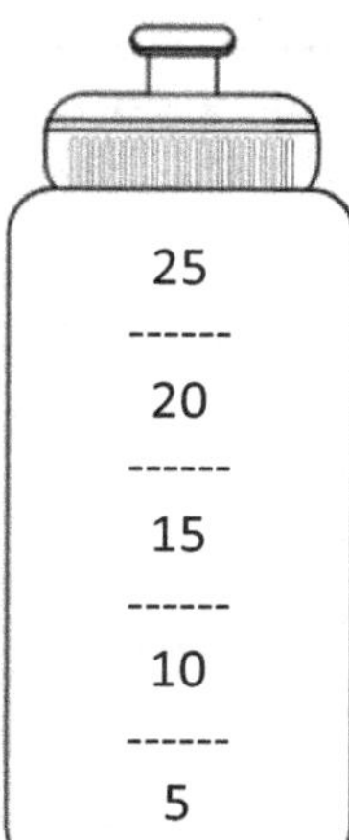

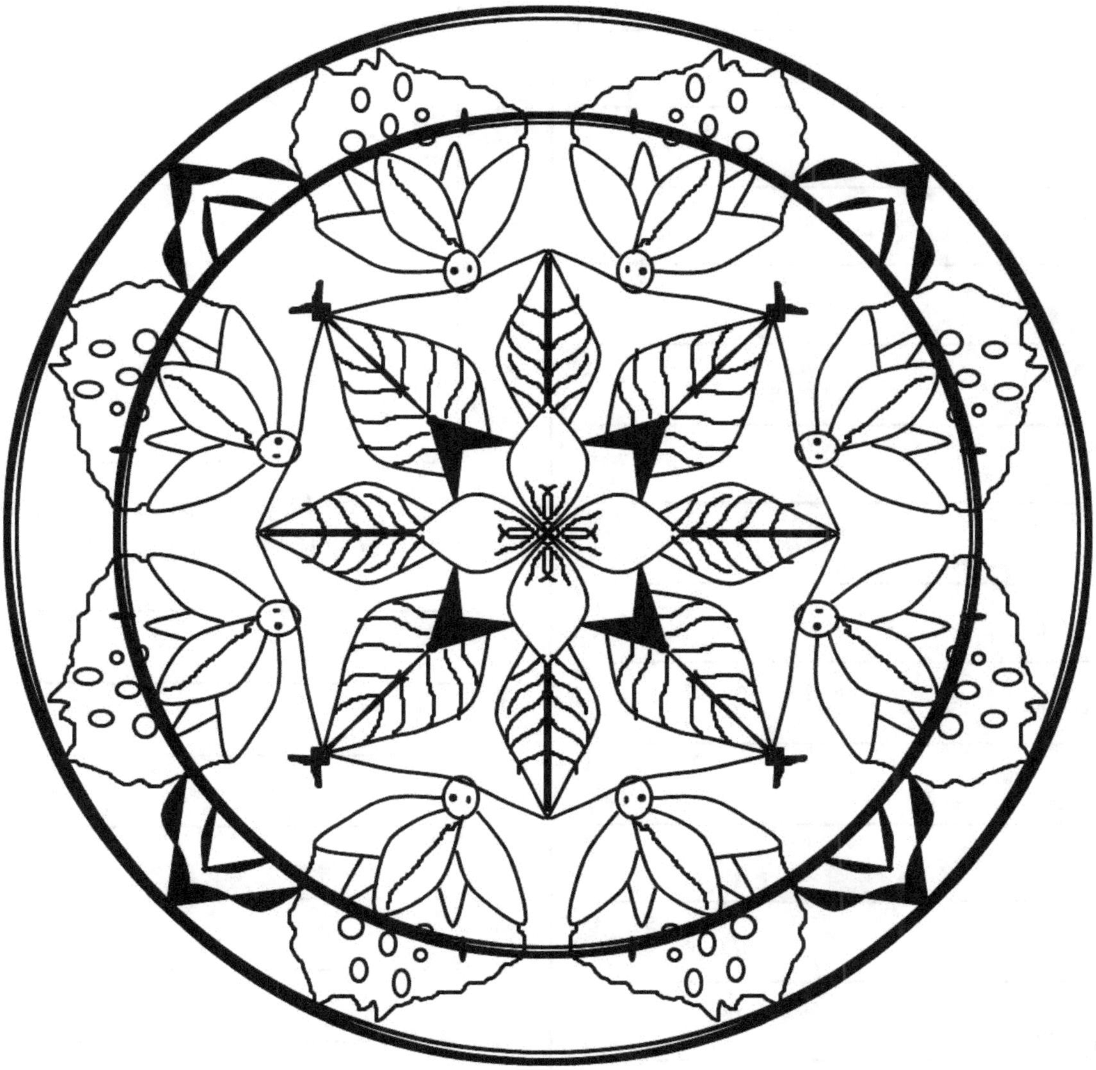

Day Eighteen _______

Time	
5:00	____________________
6:00	____________________
7:00	____________________
8:00	____________________
9:00	____________________
10:00	____________________
11:00	____________________
Noon	____________________
1:00	____________________
2:00	____________________
3:00	____________________
4:00	____________________
5:00	____________________
6:00	____________________
7:00	____________________
8:00	____________________
9:00	____________________
10:00	____________________
11:00	____________________
Midnight	____________________

Today's victories

Where will you shine your light this week?

The Training

<table>
<tr><td>Exercise</td><td>Set 1</td><td>Set 2</td><td>Set 3</td><td>Set 4</td><td>Set 5</td><td>notes</td></tr>
<tr><td></td><td></td><td></td><td></td><td></td><td></td><td></td></tr>
<tr><td></td><td></td><td></td><td></td><td></td><td></td><td></td></tr>
<tr><td></td><td></td><td></td><td></td><td></td><td></td><td></td></tr>
<tr><td></td><td></td><td></td><td></td><td></td><td></td><td></td></tr>
<tr><td></td><td></td><td></td><td></td><td></td><td></td><td></td></tr>
<tr><td></td><td></td><td></td><td></td><td></td><td></td><td></td></tr>
</table>

Time started: _____________ Time ended: _____________

Location: ____

Feelings before training:

Feelings after training

NUTRITION

Meal 1
time eaten: _________

Meal 2
time eaten: _________

Meal 3
time eaten: _________

Meal 4
time eaten: _________

Meal 5
time eaten: _________

Hydration

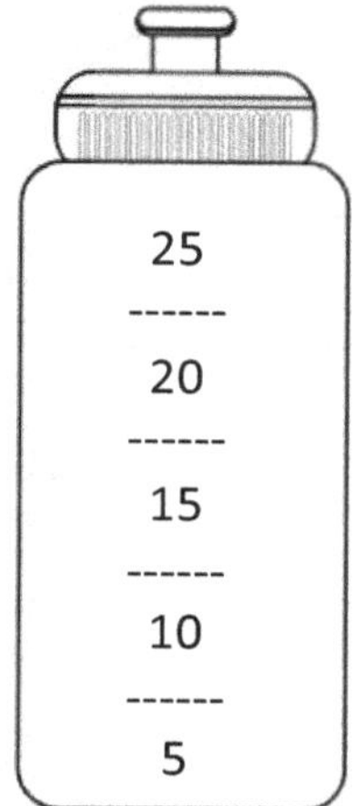 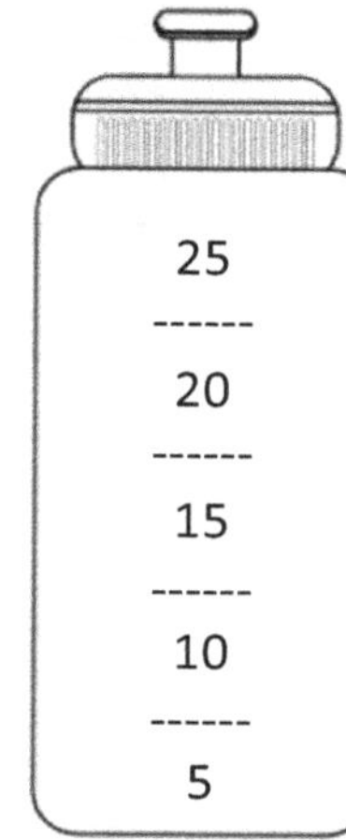 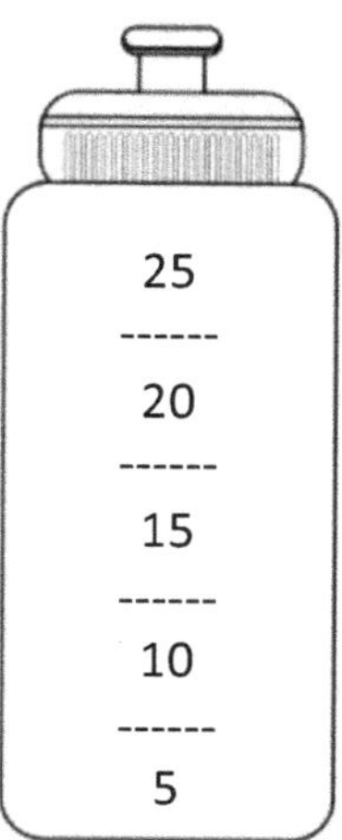 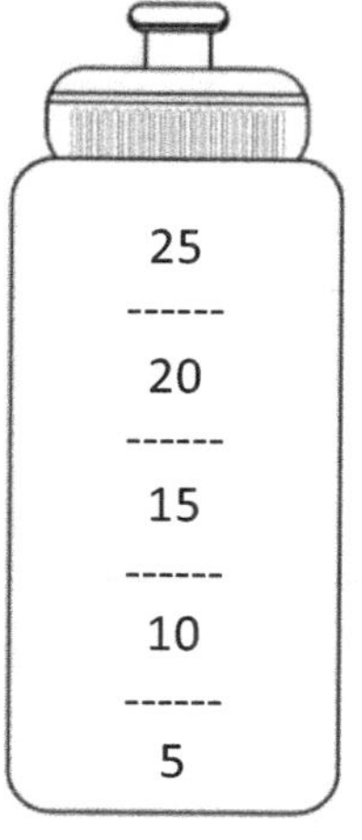 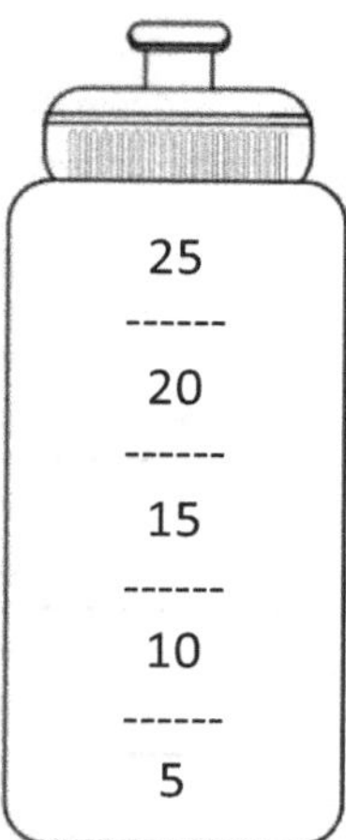

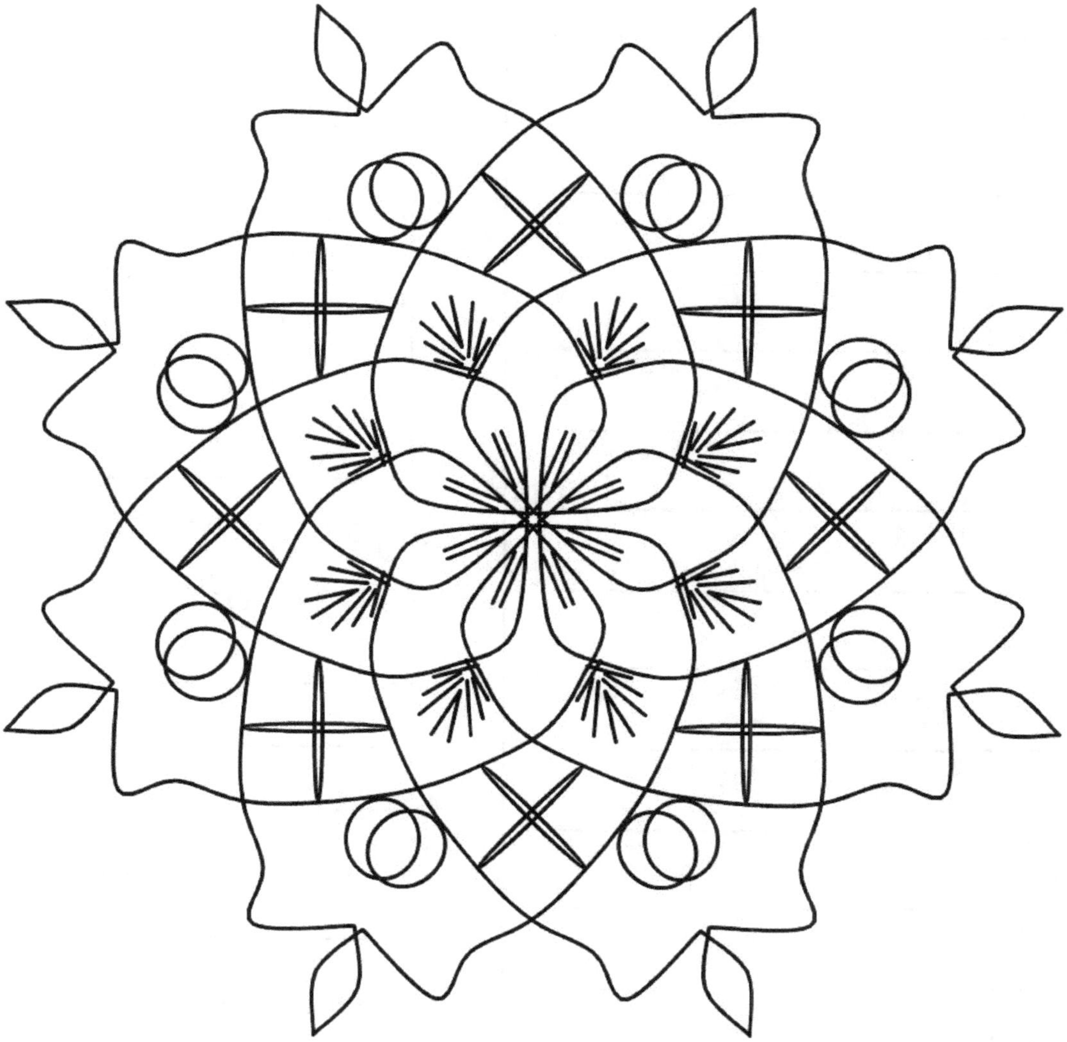

Day Nineteen _______

5:00 _______________________________

6:00 _______________________________

7:00 _______________________________

8:00 _______________________________

9:00 _______________________________

10:00 ______________________________

11:00 ______________________________

Noon _______________________________

1:00 _______________________________

2:00 _______________________________

3:00 _______________________________

4:00 _______________________________

5:00 _______________________________

6:00 _______________________________

7:00 _______________________________

8:00 _______________________________

9:00 _______________________________

10:00 ______________________________

11:00 ______________________________

Midnight ___________________________

top priorities for today

____

____

____

____

Today's victories

You are charming, how will you show it?

____

____

____

____

____

____

The Training

Exercise	Set 1	Set 2	Set 3	Set 4	Set 5	notes

Time started: _____________ Time ended: _____________

Location: ____

Feelings before training:

Feelings after training

NUTRITION

Meal 1

time eaten: _________

Meal 2

time eaten: _________

Meal 3

time eaten: _________

Meal 4

time eaten: _________

Meal 5

time eaten: _________

Hydration

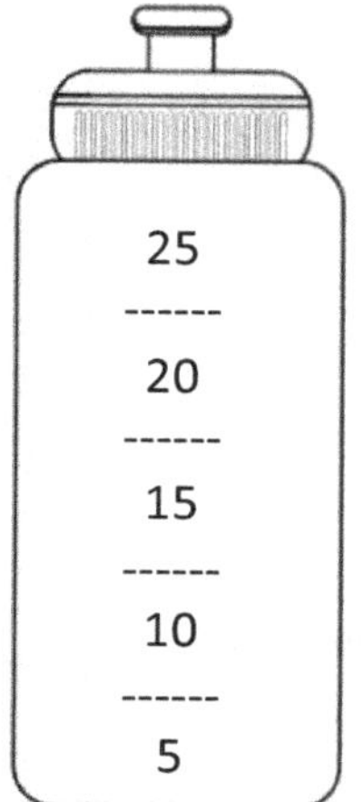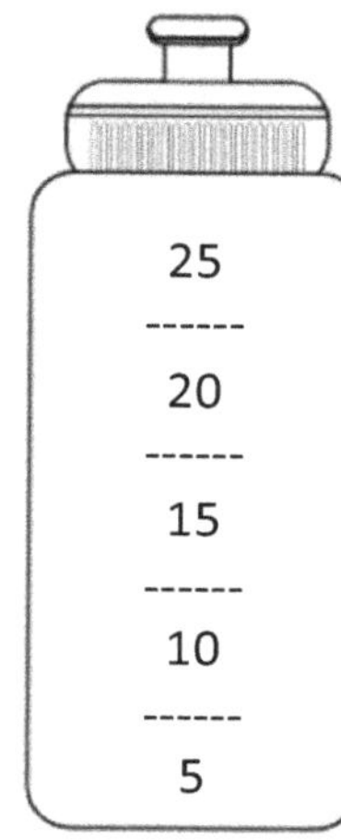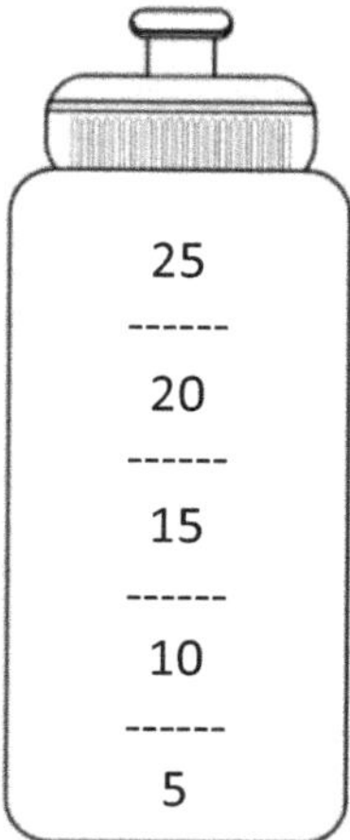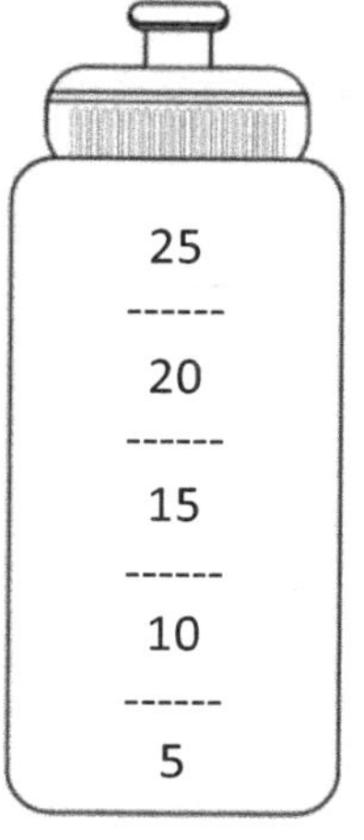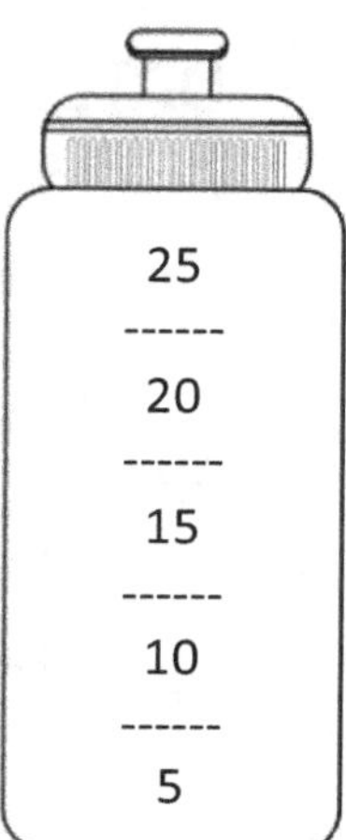

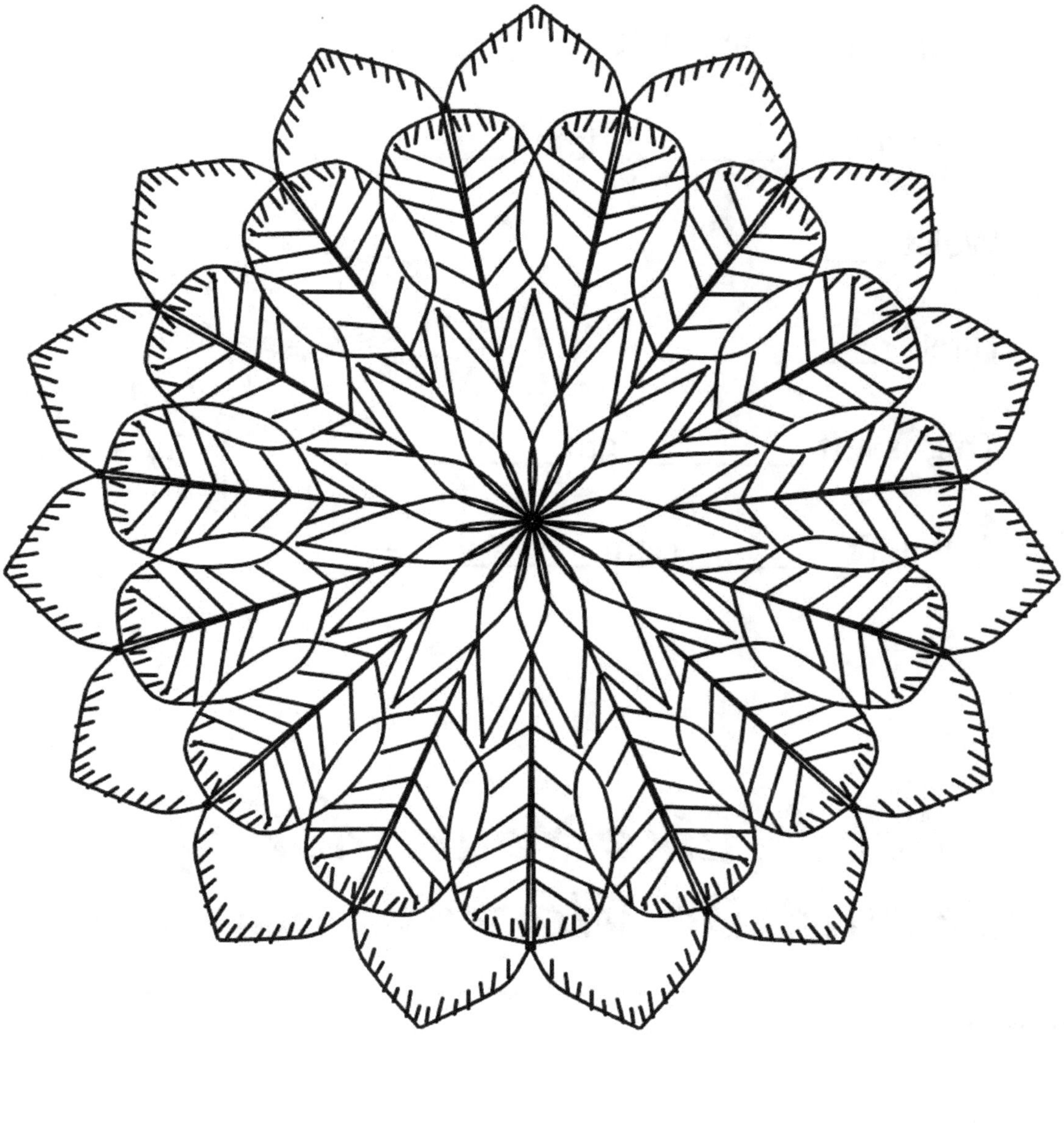

Measurements

P
R
O
G
R
E
S
S

C
H
E
C
K

DATE: _____________

Weight: _______

Neck _______

Shoulders _______

Chest _______

Bicep / upper arm left _________ right _______

Forearm left _________ right _______

Waist _______

Hips _______

Thighs left _________ right ______

Calf left _________ right _______

Food, Like Your Money,
Should Be Working For You

Day Twenty _______

5:00 _______________________

6:00 _______________________

7:00 _______________________

8:00 _______________________

9:00 _______________________

10:00 ______________________

11:00 ______________________

Noon _______________________

1:00 _______________________

2:00 _______________________

3:00 _______________________

4:00 _______________________

5:00 _______________________

6:00 _______________________

7:00 _______________________

8:00 _______________________

9:00 _______________________

10:00 ______________________

11:00 ______________________

Midnight ____________________

top priorities for today

____

____

____

____

Today's victories

What is your level of understanding difficult situations?

____

____

____

____

____

The *Stella Society* Workout

Exercise	Set 1	Set 2	Set 3	Set 4	Set 5	notes

Time started: _____________ Time ended: _______________

Location: ____

Feelings before training:

Feelings after training

NUTRITION

Meal 1

time eaten: _________

Meal 2

time eaten: _________

Meal 3

time eaten: _________

Meal 4

time eaten: _________

Meal 5

time eaten: _________

Hydration

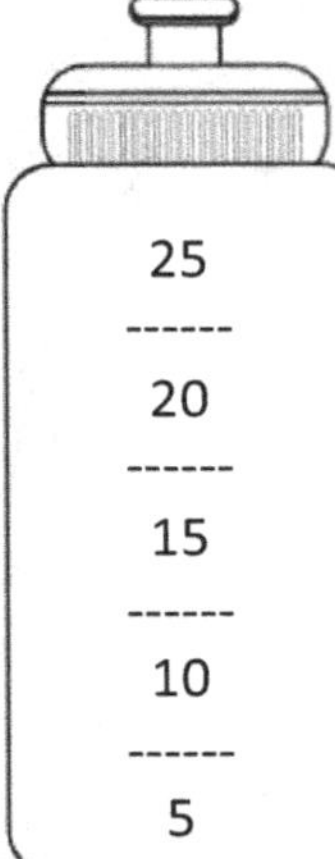

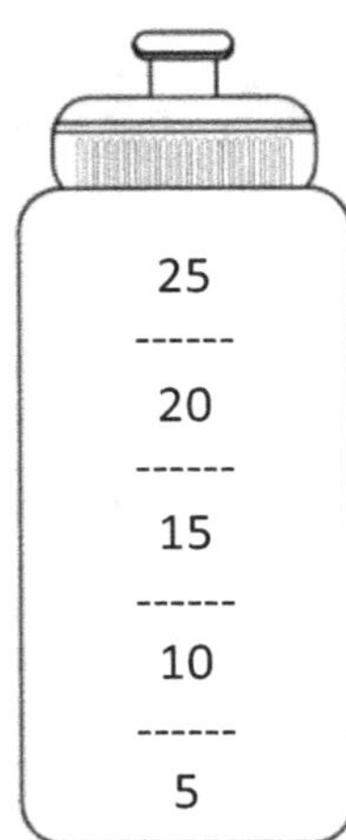

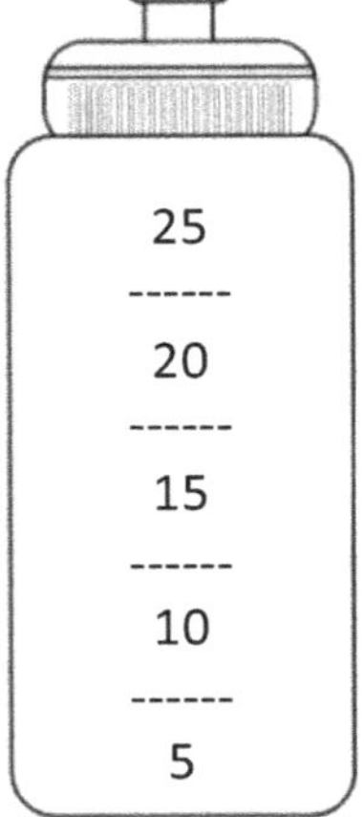

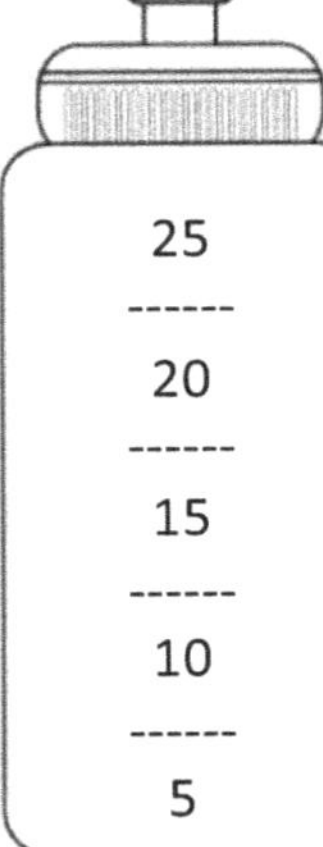

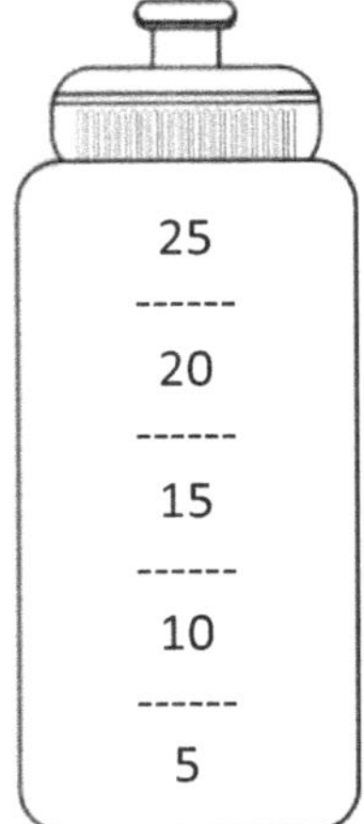

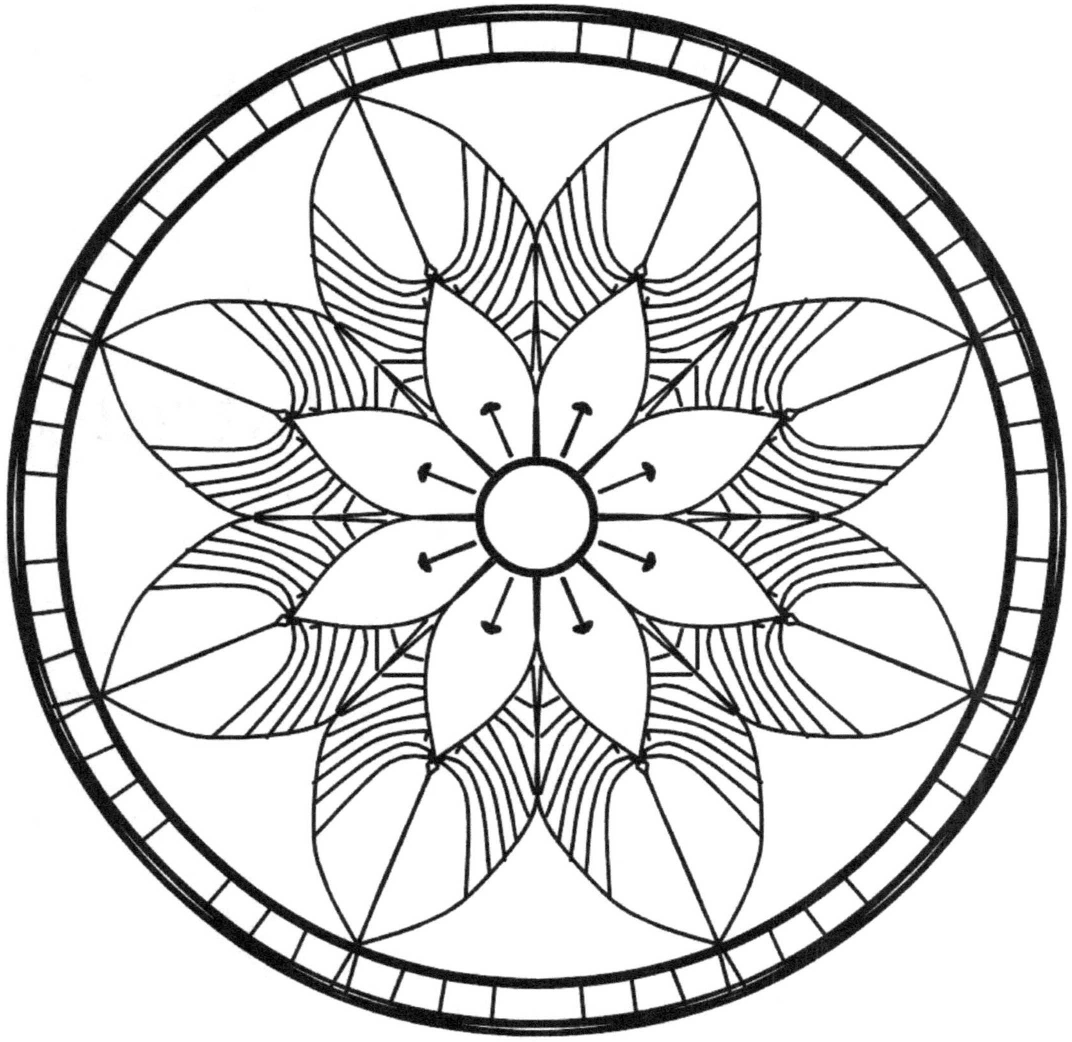

Day Twenty-one ______

Time	
5:00	______
6:00	______
7:00	______
8:00	______
9:00	______
10:00	______
11:00	______
Noon	______
1:00	______
2:00	______
3:00	______
4:00	______
5:00	______
6:00	______
7:00	______
8:00	______
9:00	______
10:00	______
11:00	______
Midnight	______

top priorities for today 🎯

Today's victories 🏆

How much can you endure?

The Stella Society Workout

Exercise	Set 1	Set 2	Set 3	Set 4	Set 5	notes

Time started: ______________   Time ended: ________________

Location: ____

Feelings before training: 🙂 😐 ☹️ 😜 😠 😟 😊 😎

Feelings after training 🙂 😐 ☹️ 😜 😠 😟 😊 😎

NUTRITION

Meal 1

time eaten: _________

Meal 2

time eaten: _________

Meal 3

time eaten: _________

Meal 4

time eaten: _________

Meal 5

time eaten: _________

Hydration

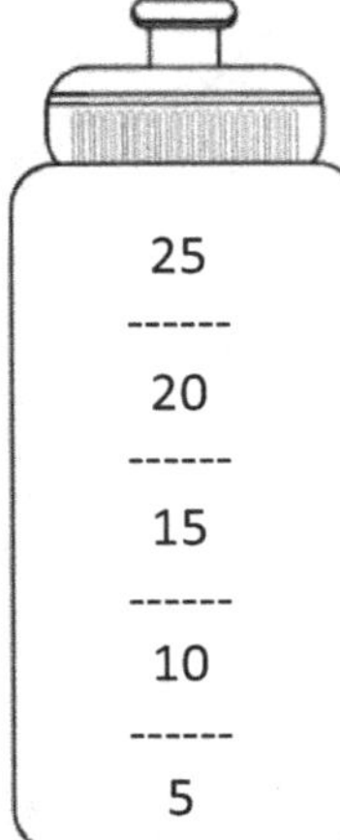
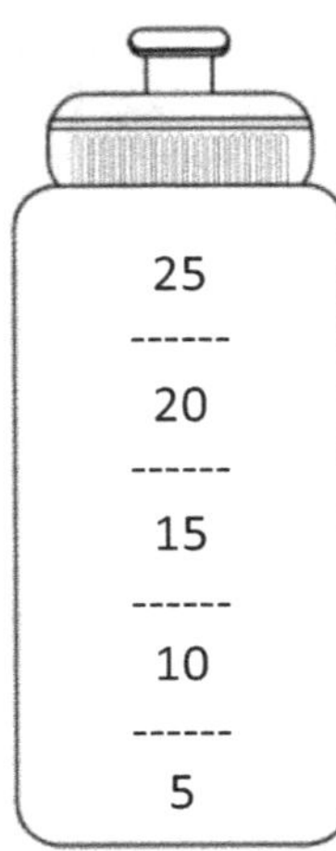
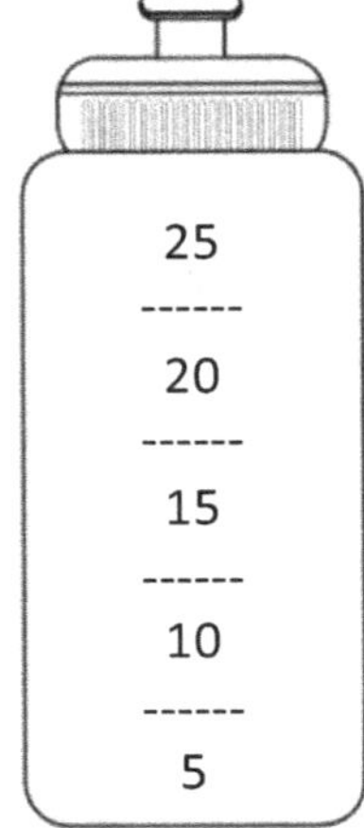
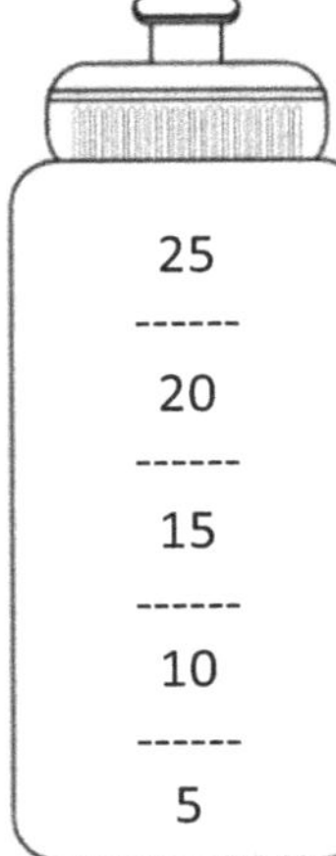
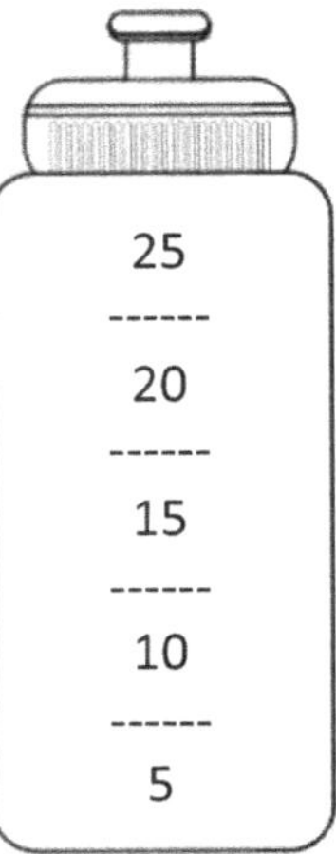

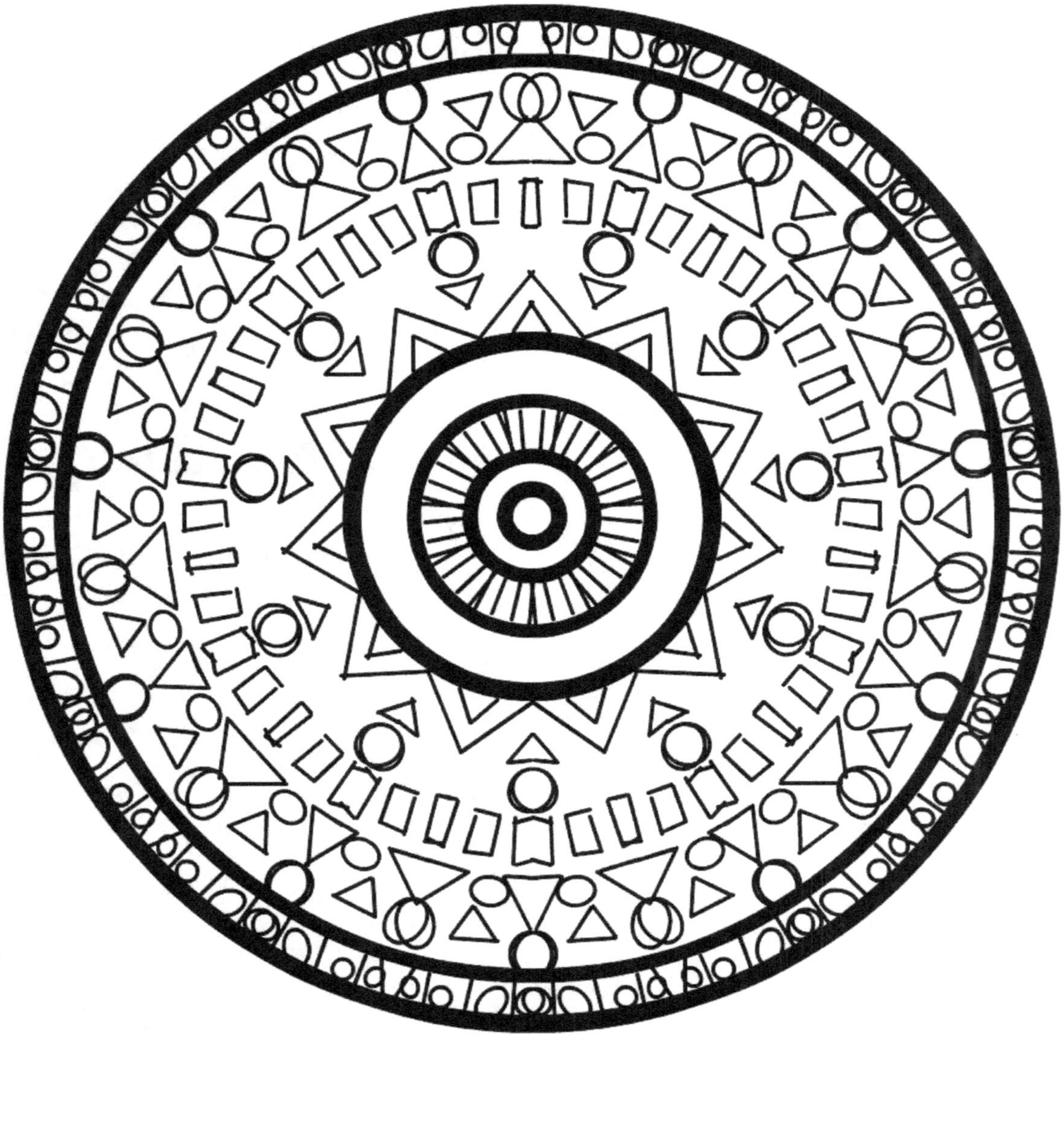

Day Twenty-two _______

5:00 _______________________________

6:00 _______________________________

7:00 _______________________________

8:00 _______________________________

9:00 _______________________________

10:00 ______________________________

11:00 ______________________________

Noon _______________________________

1:00 _______________________________

2:00 _______________________________

3:00 _______________________________

4:00 _______________________________

5:00 _______________________________

6:00 _______________________________

7:00 _______________________________

8:00 _______________________________

9:00 _______________________________

10:00 ______________________________

11:00 ______________________________

Midnight ____________________

top priorities for today

____

____

____

____

Today's victories

List 5 ways to be thoughtful.

____

____

____

____

____

The Stella Society Workout

Exercise	Set 1	Set 2	Set 3	Set 4	Set 5	notes

Time started: _____________ Time ended: _______________

Location: ____

Feelings before training:

Feelings after training

NUTRITION

Meal 1
time eaten: _________

Meal 2
time eaten: _________

Meal 3
time eaten: _________

Meal 4
time eaten: _________

Meal 5
time eaten: _________

Hydration

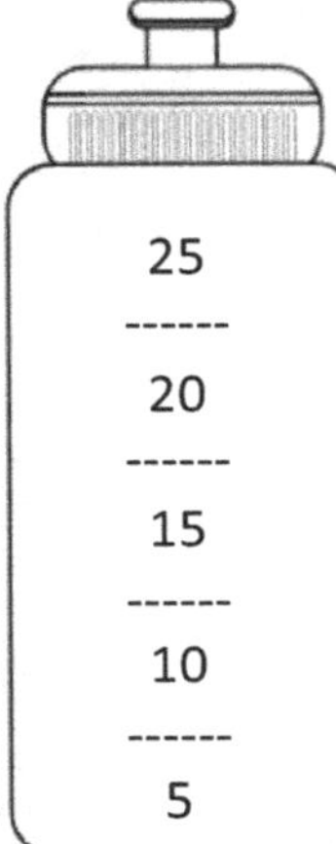 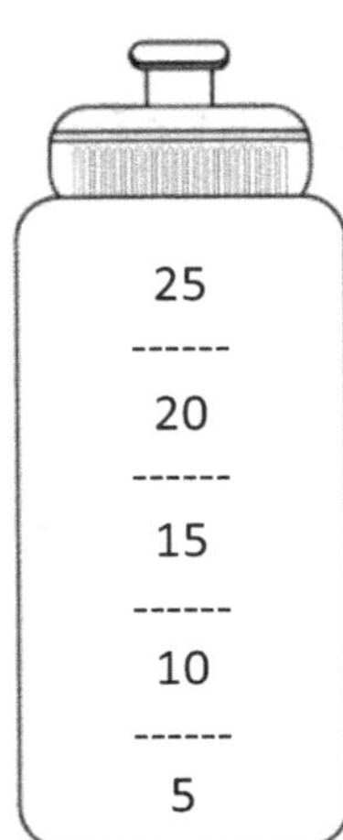 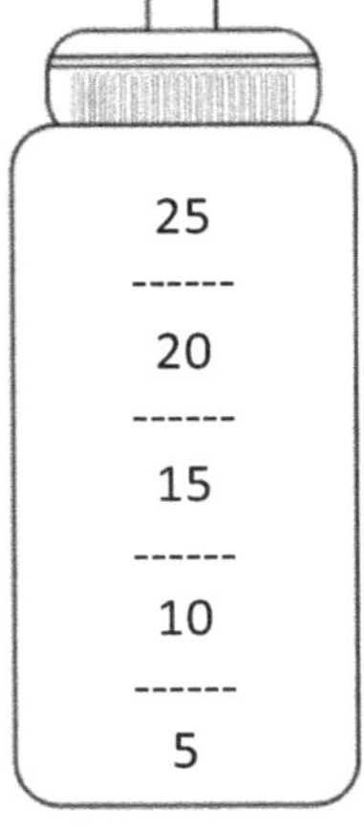 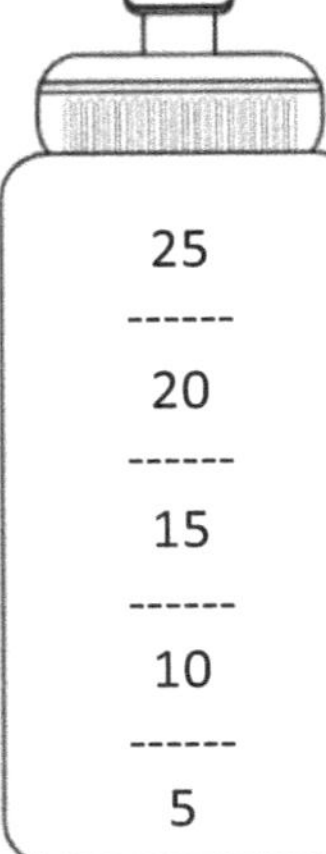 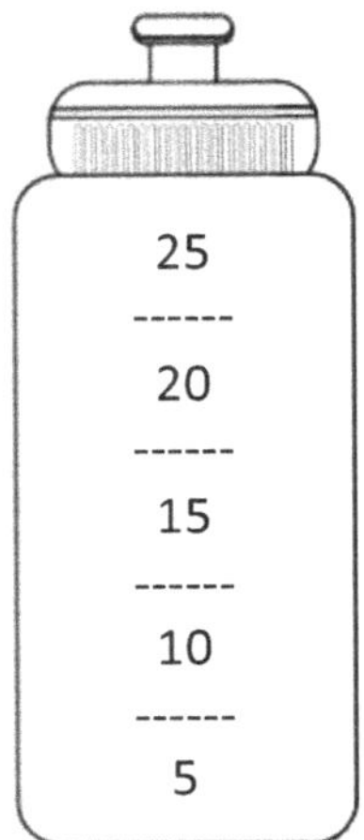

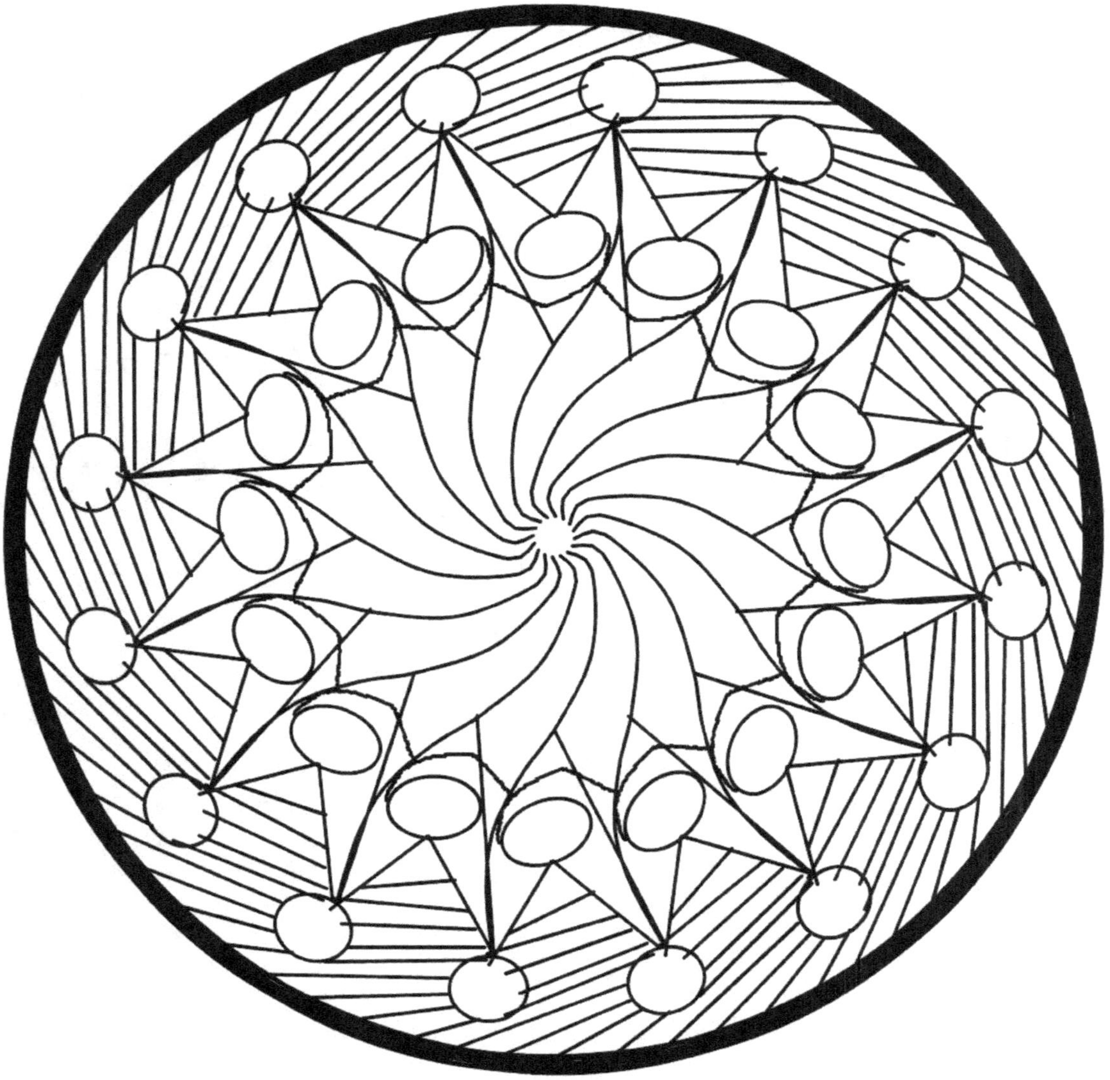

Day Twenty-three _______

5:00 _____________	
6:00 _____________	
7:00 _____________	
8:00 _____________	
9:00 _____________	
10:00 _____________	
11:00 _____________	
Noon _____________	
1:00 _____________	
2:00 _____________	
3:00 _____________	
4:00 _____________	
5:00 _____________	
6:00 _____________	
7:00 _____________	
8:00 _____________	
9:00 _____________	
10:00 _____________	
11:00 _____________	
Midnight _____________	

top priorities for today

____

____

____

____

____

Today's victories

Why should you be unapologetic?

____

____

____

____

____

____

The Stella Society Workout

Exercise	Set 1	Set 2	Set 3	Set 4	Set 5	notes

Time started: ______________ Time ended: ______________

Location: ____

Feelings before training:

Feelings after training

NUTRITION

Meal 1
time eaten: _________

Meal 2
time eaten: _________

Meal 3
time eaten: _________

Meal 4
time eaten: _________

Meal 5
time eaten: _________

Hydration

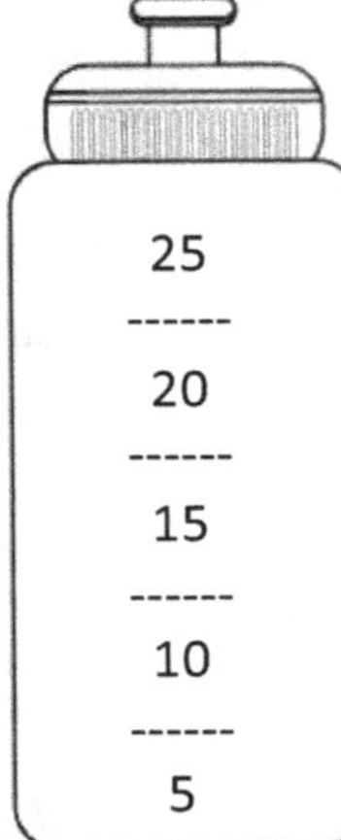

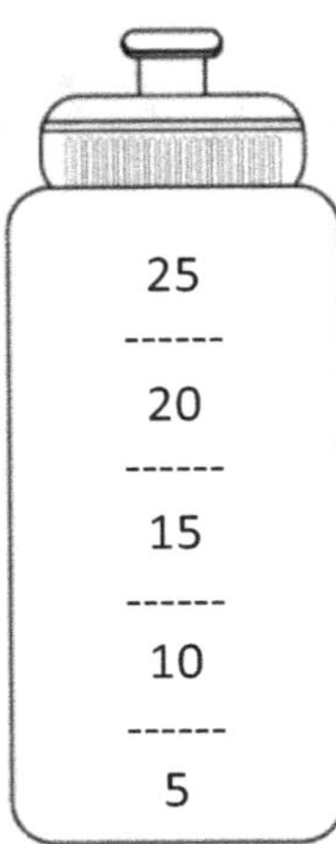

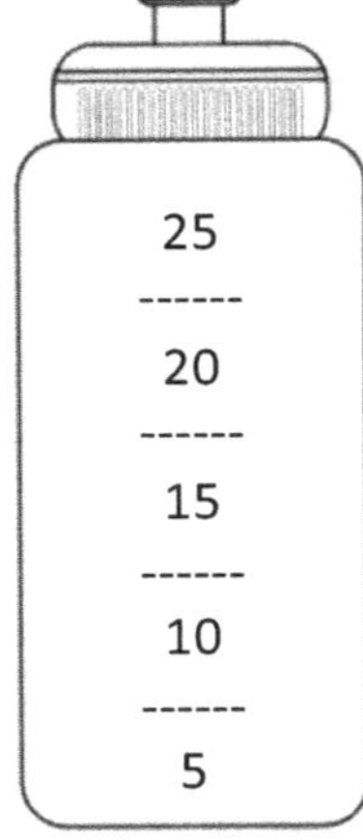

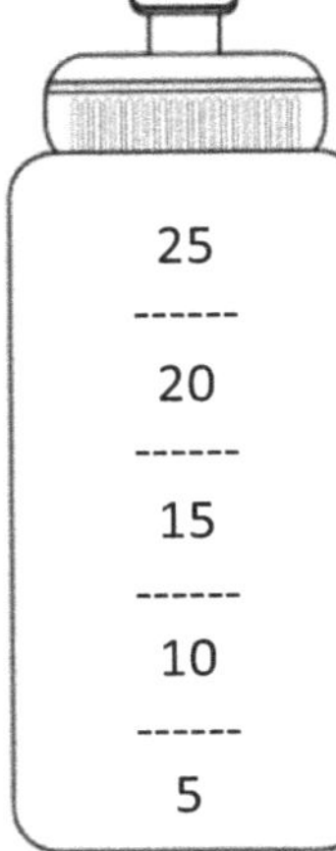

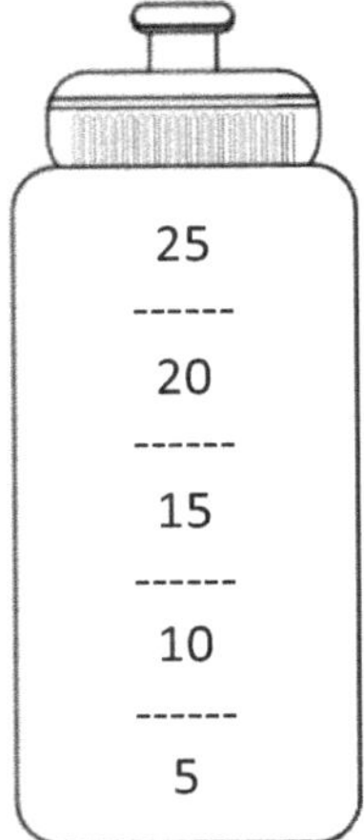

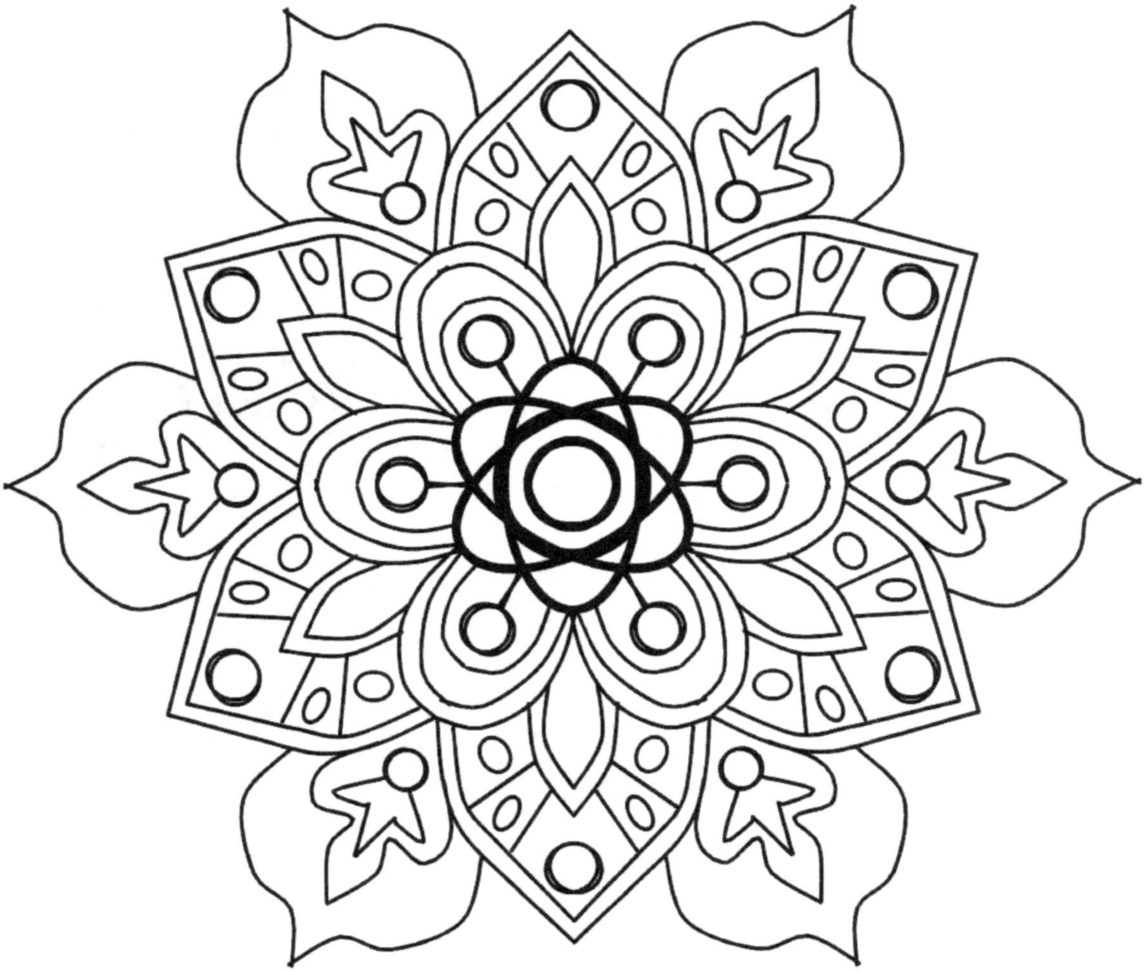

Day Twenty-four ______

Time	
5:00	______________
6:00	______________
7:00	______________
8:00	______________
9:00	______________
10:00	_____________
11:00	_____________
Noon	______________
1:00	______________
2:00	______________
3:00	______________
4:00	______________
5:00	______________
6:00	______________
7:00	______________
8:00	______________
9:00	______________
10:00	_____________
11:00	_____________
Midnight	___________

Today's victories

What can you set on fire
with your fierceness?

The Stella Society Workout

Exercise	Set 1	Set 2	Set 3	Set 4	Set 5	notes

Time started: _____________   Time ended: ______________

Location: ____

Feelings before training:

Feelings after training

NUTRITION

Meal 1

time eaten: _________

Meal 2

time eaten: _________

Meal 3

time eaten: _________

Meal 4

time eaten: _________

Meal 5

time eaten: _________

Hydration

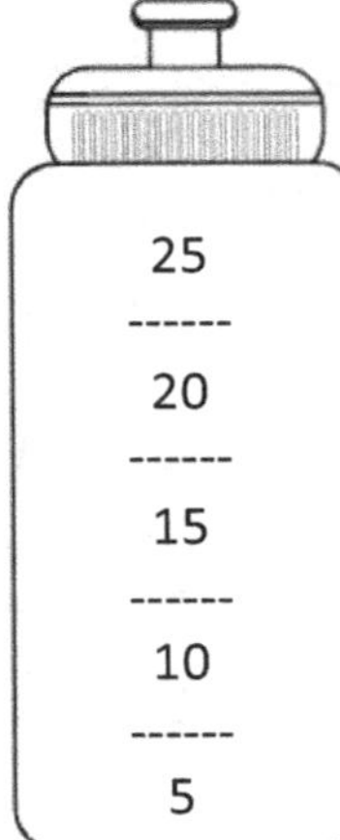
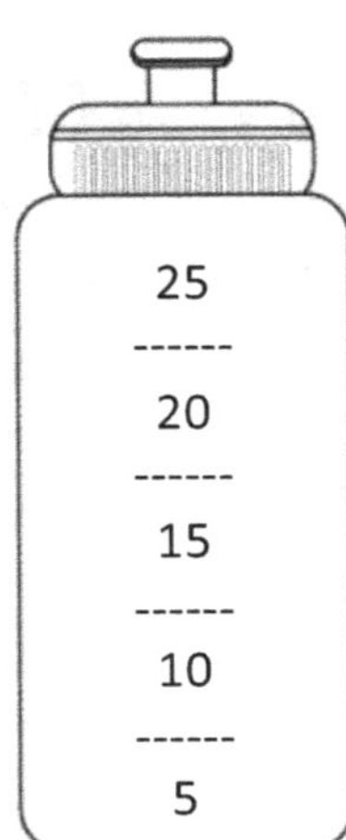
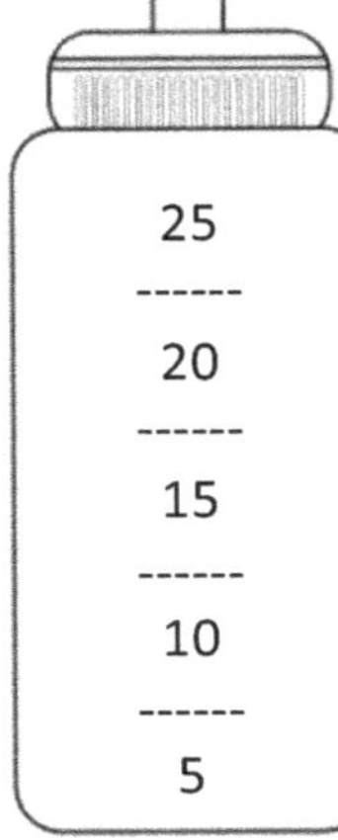
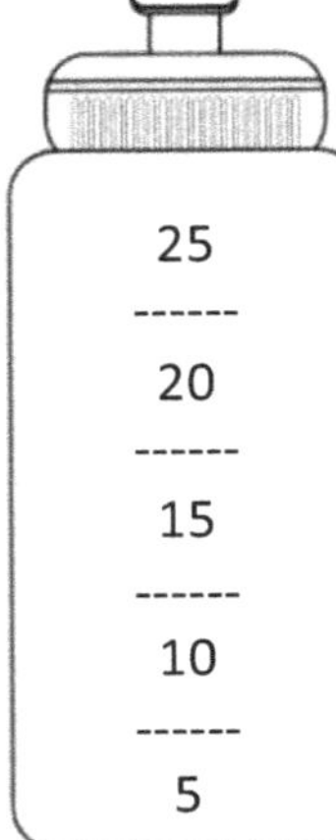
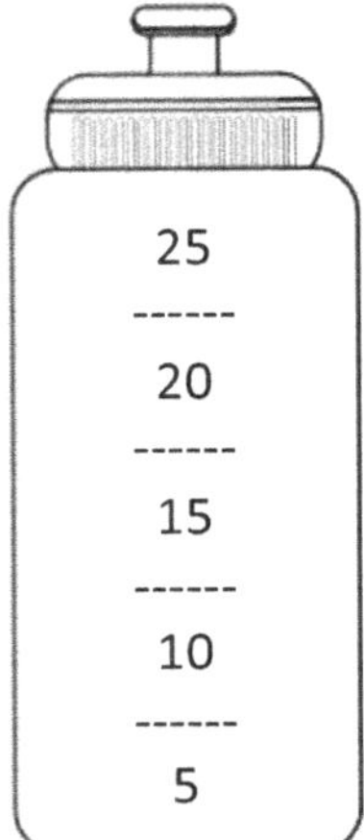

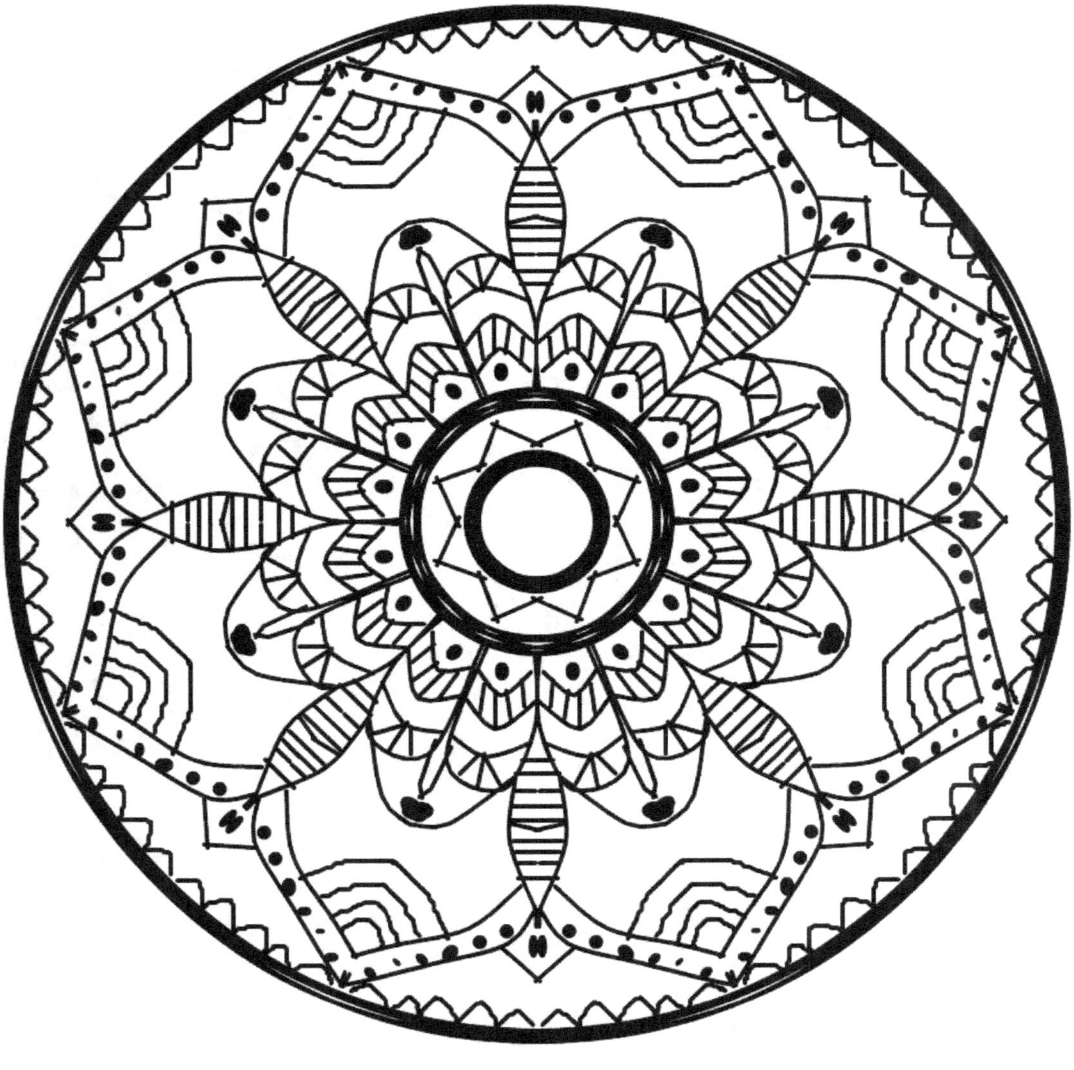

Day Twenty-five _______

5:00 _______________________

6:00 _______________________

7:00 _______________________

8:00 _______________________

9:00 _______________________

10:00 _______________________

11:00 _______________________

Noon _______________________

1:00 _______________________

2:00 _______________________

3:00 _______________________

4:00 _______________________

5:00 _______________________

6:00 _______________________

7:00 _______________________

8:00 _______________________

9:00 _______________________

10:00 _______________________

11:00 _______________________

Midnight _______________________

top priorities for today

____
____
____
____
____

Today's victories

Make it your mission to stay positive. Write your positive mission statement.

____
____
____
____
____

The ⟨Stella Society⟩ Workout

Exercise	Set 1	Set 2	Set 3	Set 4	Set 5	notes

Time started: _____________   Time ended: _______________

Location: ____

Feelings before training: 🙂 😑 🙁 😜 😠 😒 😊 😎

Feelings after training 🙂 😑 🙁 😜 😠 😒 😊 😎

NUTRITION

Meal 1
time eaten: _________

Meal 2
time eaten: _________

Meal 3
time eaten: _________

Meal 4
time eaten: _________

Meal 5
time eaten: _________

Hydration

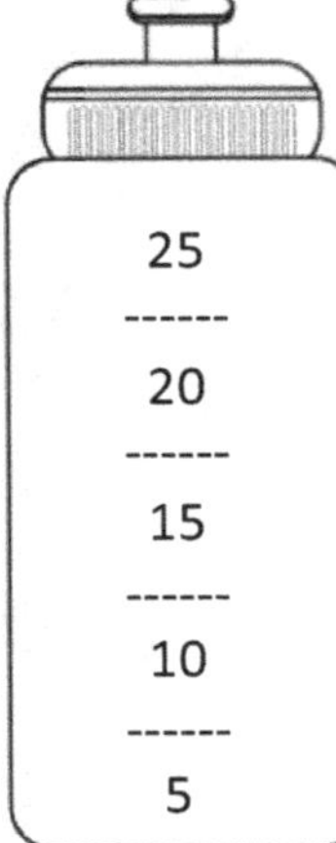

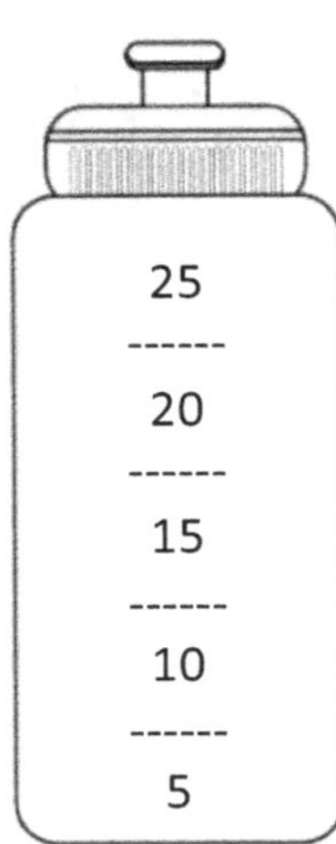

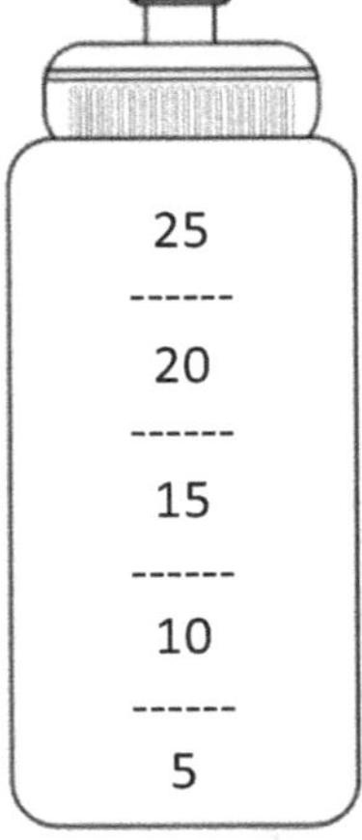

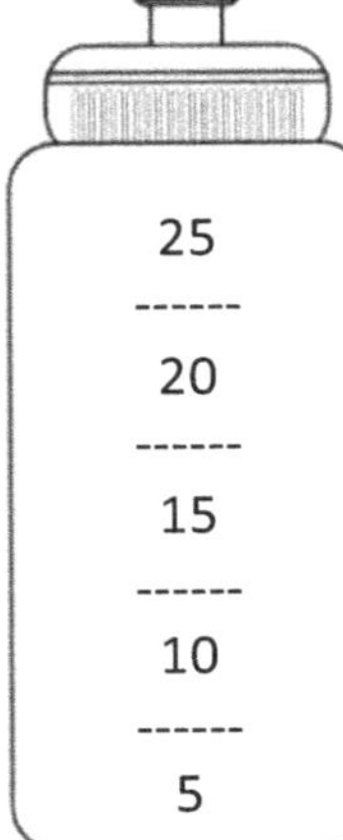

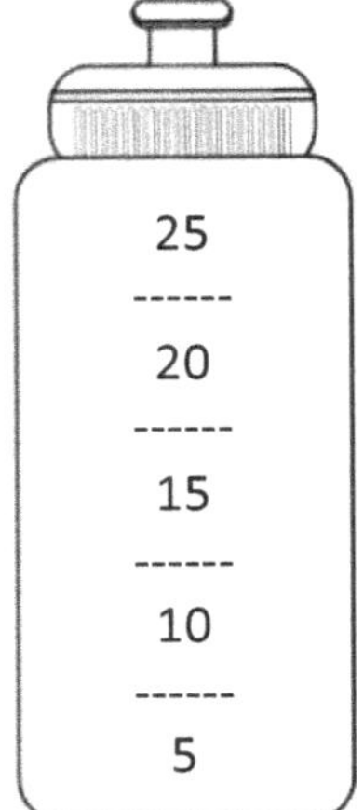

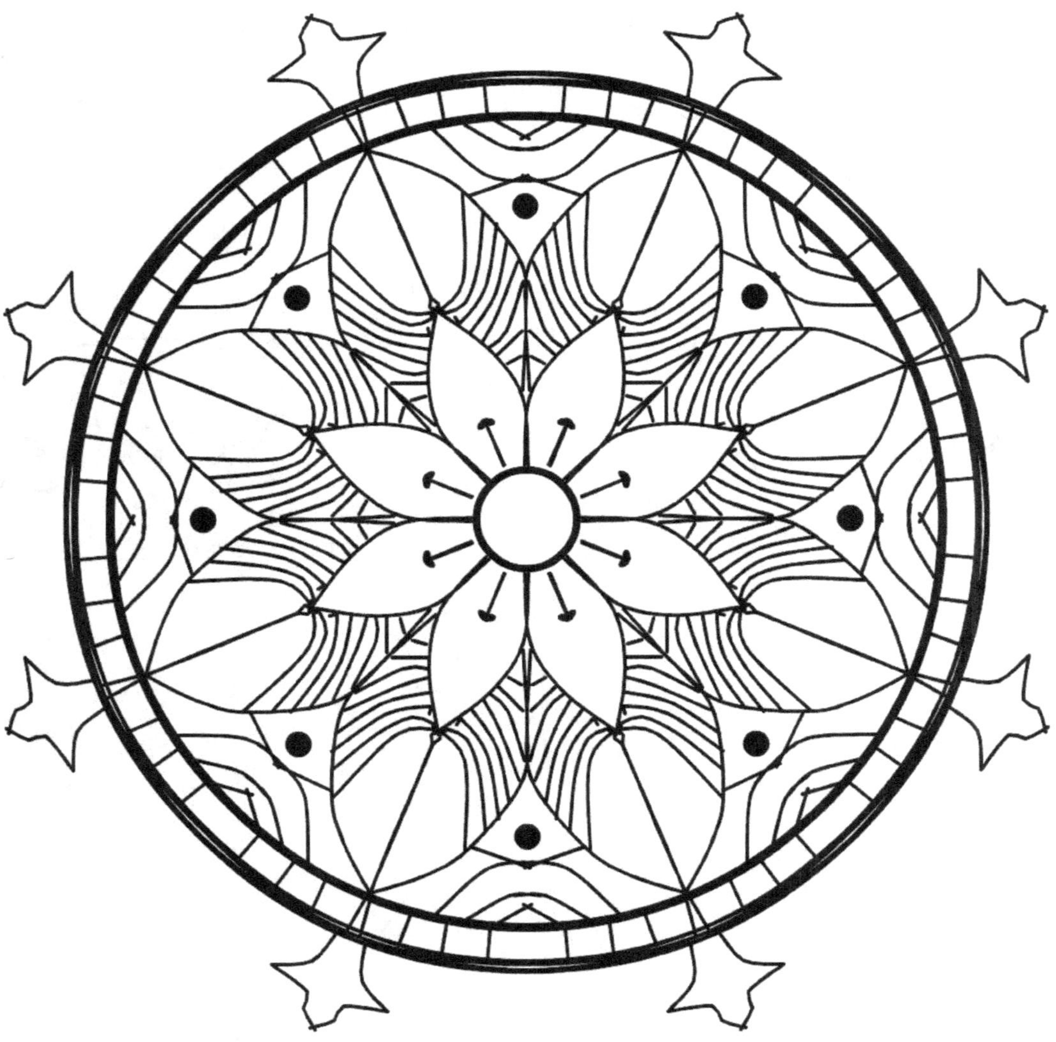

Day Twenty-six _______

<table>
<tr><td valign="top">

5:00 _______________

6:00 _______________

7:00 _______________

8:00 _______________

9:00 _______________

10:00 ______________

11:00 ______________

Noon _______________

1:00 _______________

2:00 _______________

3:00 _______________

4:00 _______________

5:00 _______________

6:00 _______________

7:00 _______________

8:00 _______________

9:00 _______________

10:00 ______________

11:00 ______________

Midnight ___________

</td><td valign="top">

top priorities for today 🎯

____

____

____

____

Today's victories 🏆

What give you your inner energy?

____

____

____

____

____

____

____

</td></tr>
</table>

The *Stella Society* Workout

Exercise	Set 1	Set 2	Set 3	Set 4	Set 5	notes

Time started: _____________ Time ended: _____________

Location: ____

Feelings before training:

Feelings after training

NUTRITION

Meal 1

time eaten: _________

Meal 2

time eaten: _________

Meal 3

time eaten: _________

Meal 4

time eaten: _________

Meal 5

time eaten: _________

Hydration

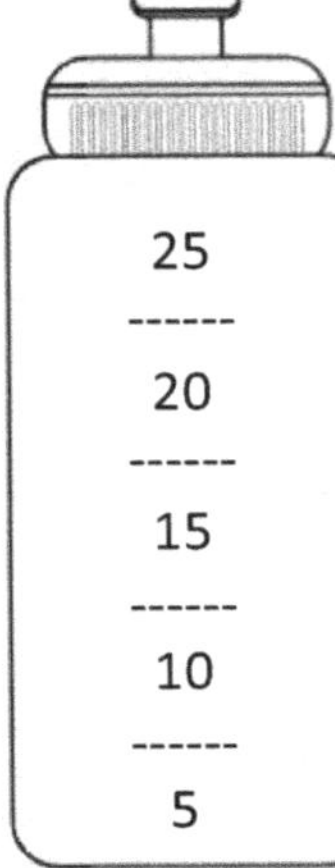
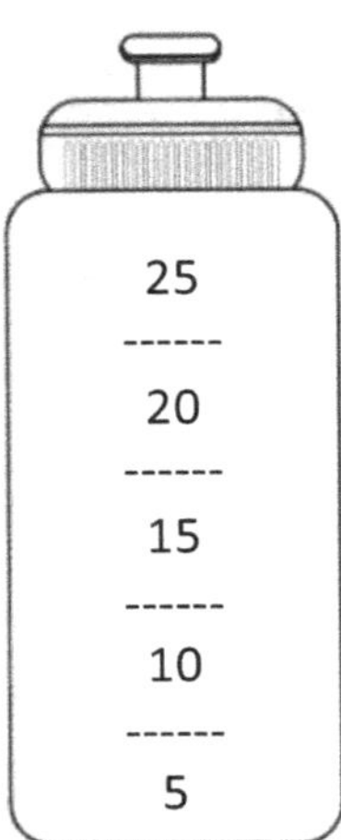
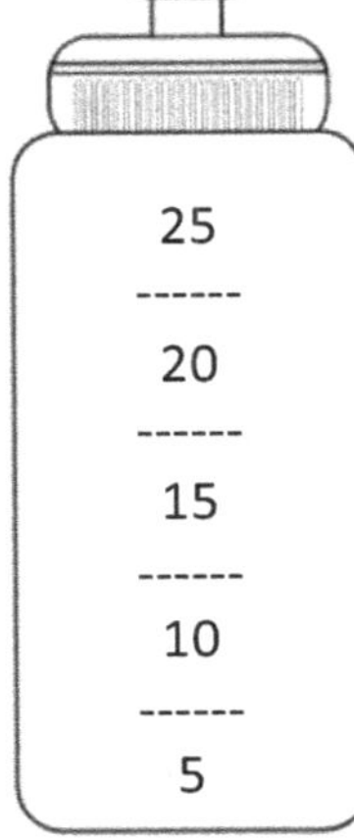
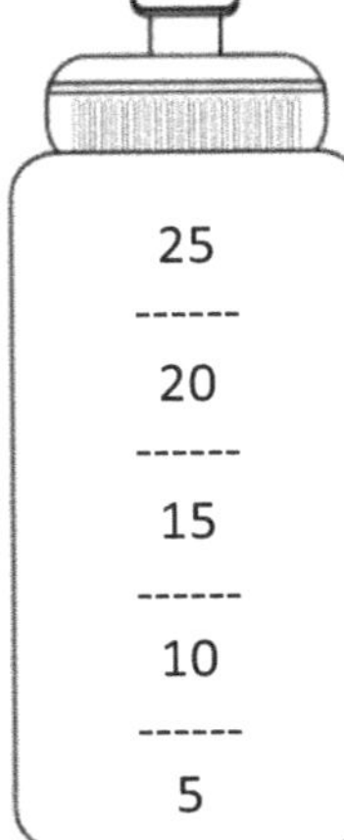
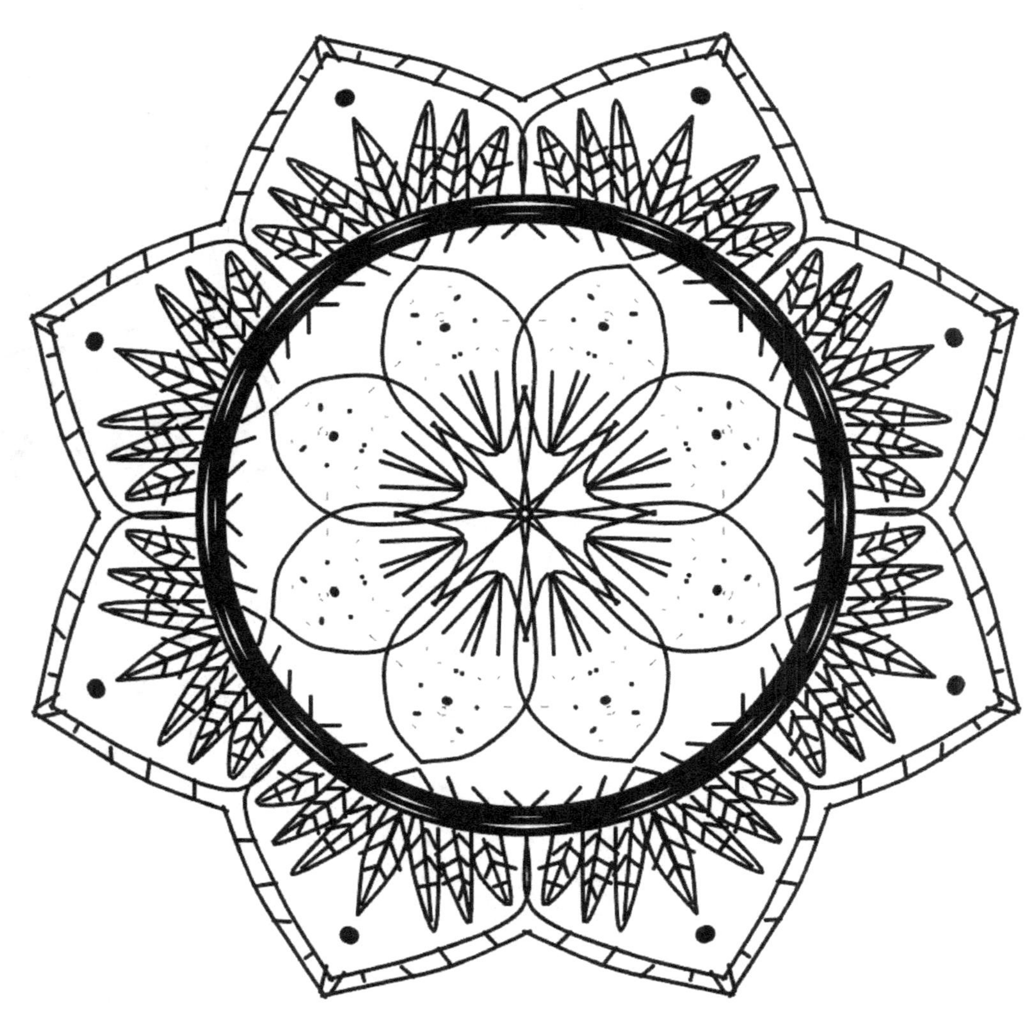

Day Twenty-seven _______

5:00 _______________________

6:00 _______________________

7:00 _______________________

8:00 _______________________

9:00 _______________________

10:00 ______________________

11:00 ______________________

Noon _______________________

1:00 _______________________

2:00 _______________________

3:00 _______________________

4:00 _______________________

5:00 _______________________

6:00 _______________________

7:00 _______________________

8:00 _______________________

9:00 _______________________

10:00 ______________________

11:00 ______________________

Midnight ___________________

top priorities for today

____

____

____

____

Today's victories

What have you stopped, but won't stop again?

____

____

____

____

____

____

____

The *Stella Society* Workout

Exercise	Set 1	Set 2	Set 3	Set 4	Set 5	notes

Time started: _____________ Time ended: _______________

Location: ____

Feelings before training: 😊 😐 🙁 😜 😠 😧 😇 😎

Feelings after training 😊 😐 🙁 😜 😠 😧 😇 😎

NUTRITION

Meal 1

time eaten: _________

Meal 2

time eaten: _________

Meal 3

time eaten: _________

Meal 4

time eaten: _________

Meal 5

time eaten: _________

Hydration

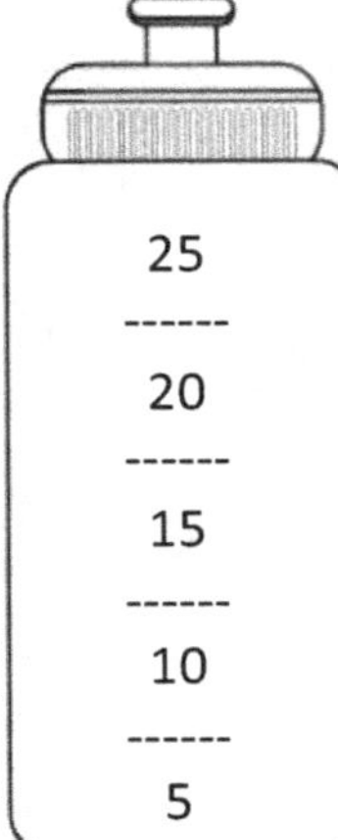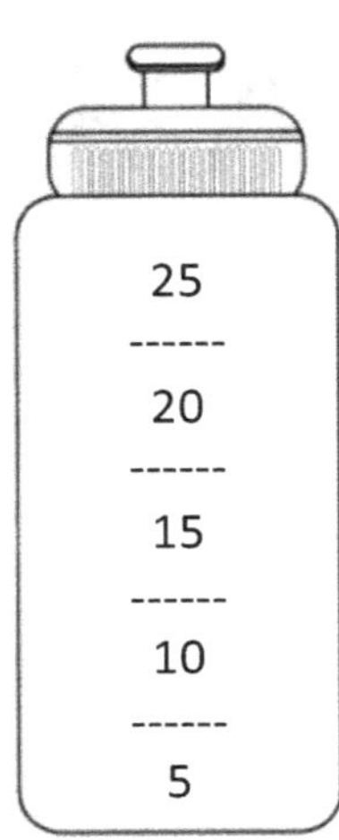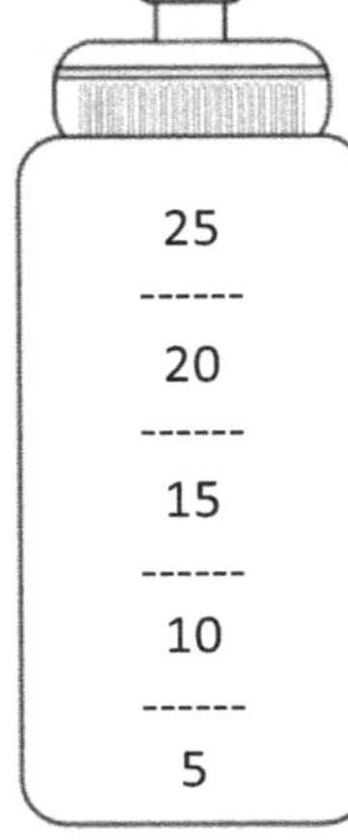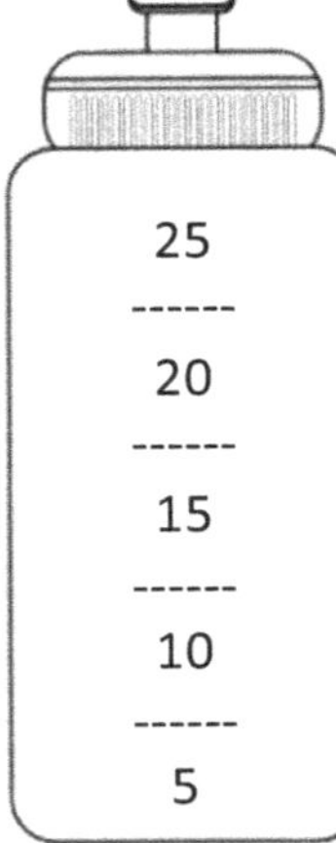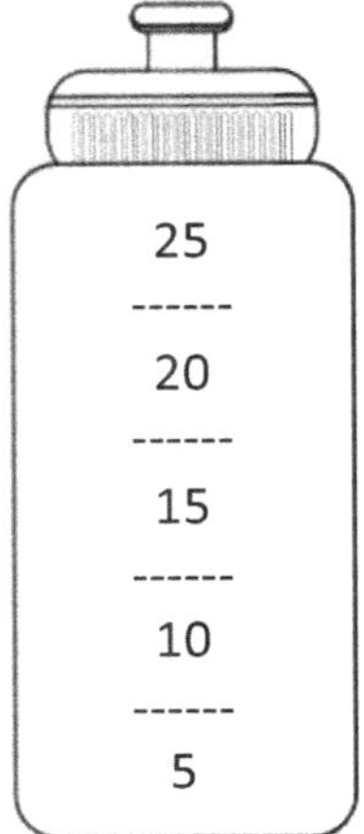

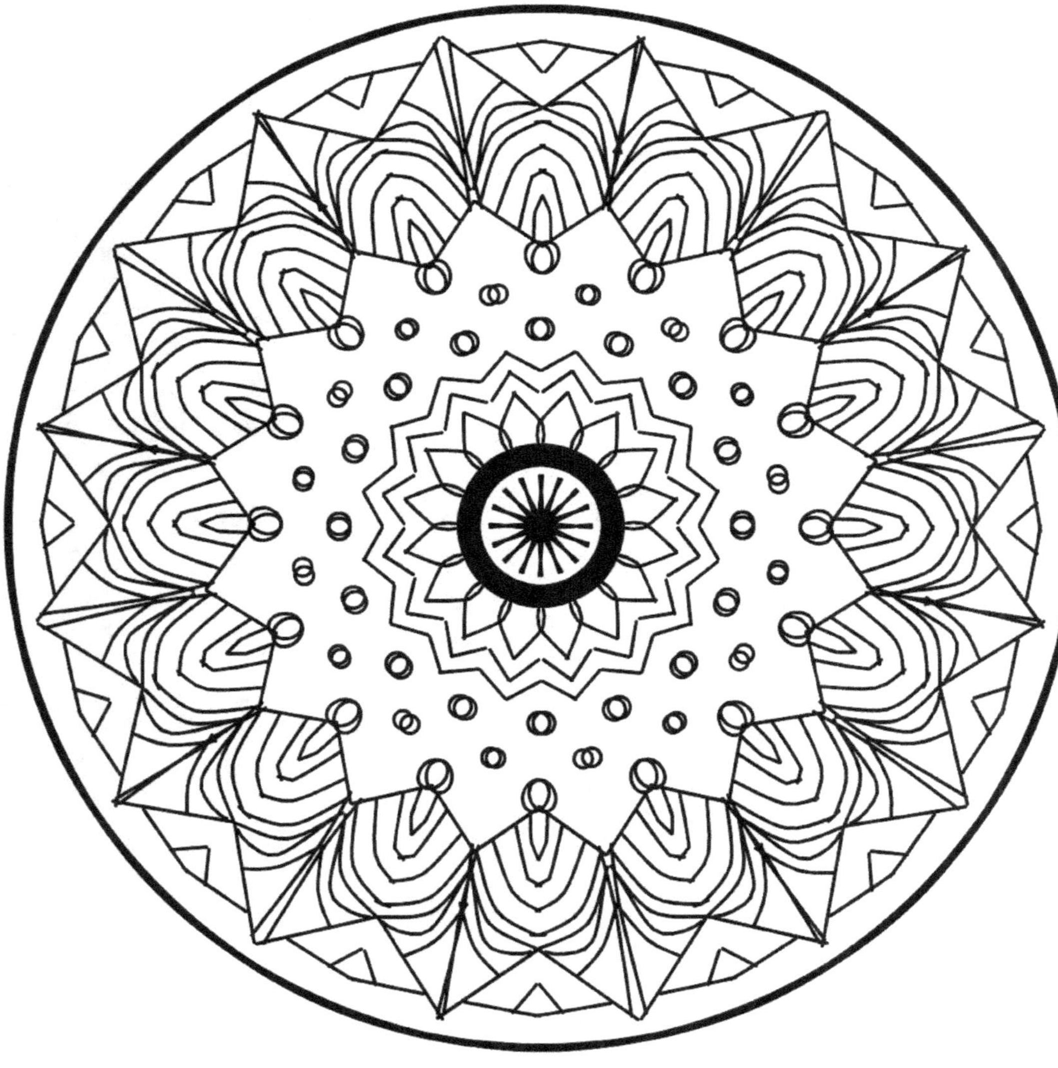

Day Twenty-eight _______

5:00 _______________________

6:00 _______________________

7:00 _______________________

8:00 _______________________

9:00 _______________________

10:00 _______________________

11:00 _______________________

Noon _______________________

1:00 _______________________

2:00 _______________________

3:00 _______________________

4:00 _______________________

5:00 _______________________

6:00 _______________________

7:00 _______________________

8:00 _______________________

9:00 _______________________

10:00 _______________________

11:00 _______________________

Midnight _______________________

top priorities for today

____

____

____

____

____

Today's victories

How do identify with being
a unicorn?

____

____

____

____

____

____

The *Stella Society* Workout

Exercise	Set 1	Set 2	Set 3	Set 4	Set 5	notes

Time started: ______________ Time ended: ______________

Location: ____

Feelings before training:

Feelings after training

NUTRITION

Meal 1
time eaten: _________

Meal 2
time eaten: _________

Meal 3
time eaten: _________

Meal 4
time eaten: _________

Meal 5
time eaten: _________

Hydration

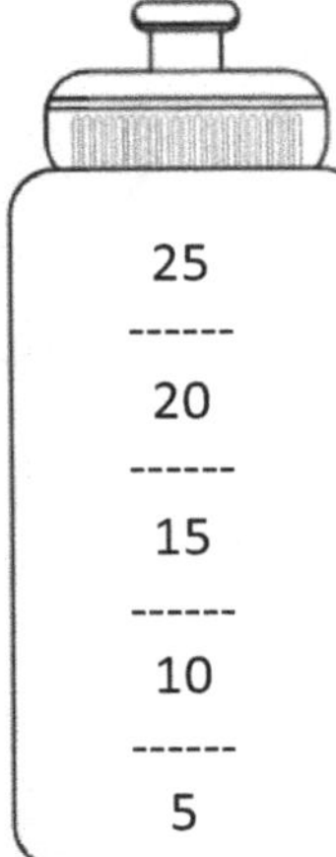

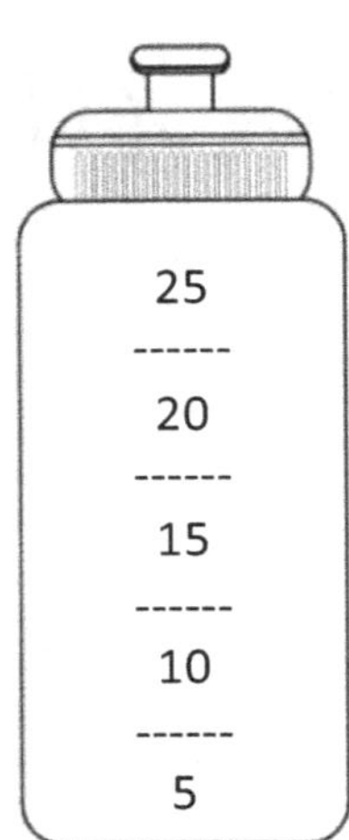

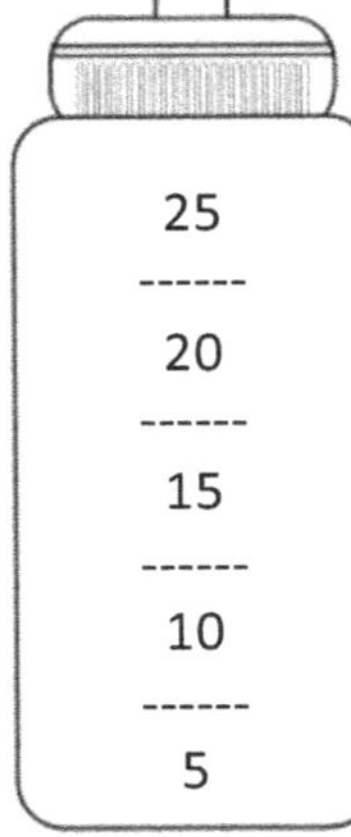

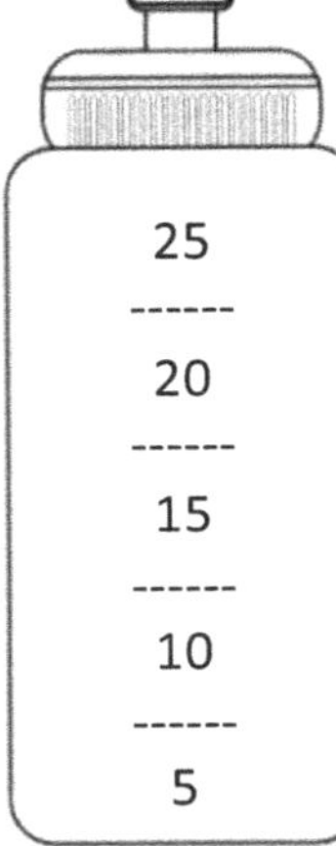

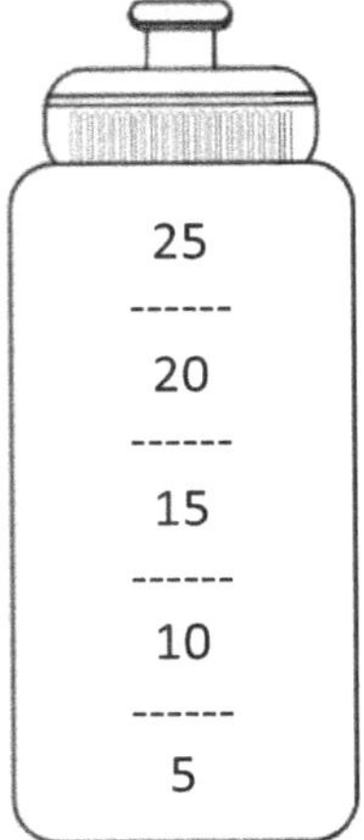

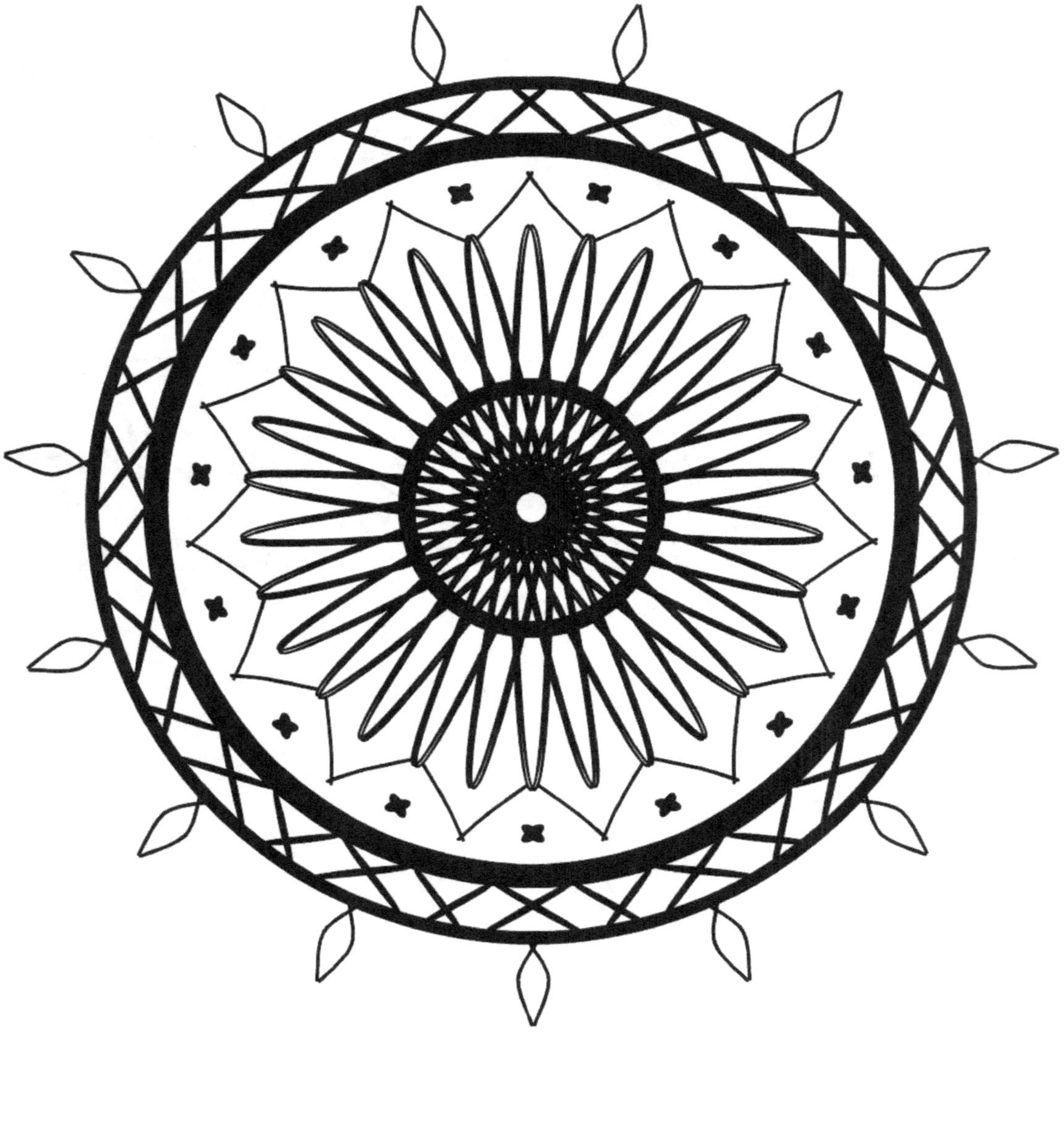

Day Twenty-nine _______

5:00 _______________________

6:00 _______________________

7:00 _______________________

8:00 _______________________

9:00 _______________________

10:00 ______________________

11:00 ______________________

Noon _______________________

1:00 _______________________

2:00 _______________________

3:00 _______________________

4:00 _______________________

5:00 _______________________

6:00 _______________________

7:00 _______________________

8:00 _______________________

9:00 _______________________

10:00 ______________________

11:00 ______________________

Midnight ___________________

top priorities for today 🎯

____

____

____

____

Today's victories 🏆

You have permission to be a
savage. What do you do with it?

____

____

____

____

____

The *Stella Society* Workout

Exercise	Set 1	Set 2	Set 3	Set 4	Set 5	notes

Time started: ______________   Time ended: ______________

Location: ____

Feelings before training:

Feelings after training

NUTRITION

Meal 1

time eaten: _________

Meal 2

time eaten: _________

Meal 3

time eaten: _________

Meal 4

time eaten: _________

Meal 5

time eaten: _________

Hydration

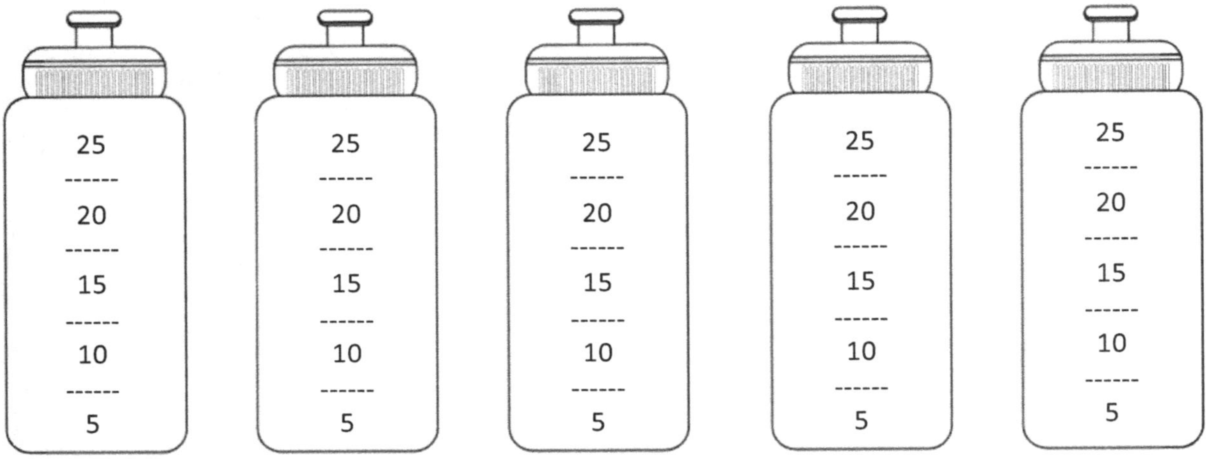

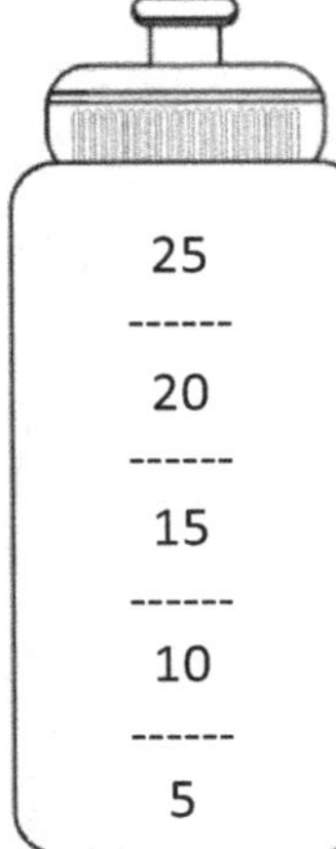 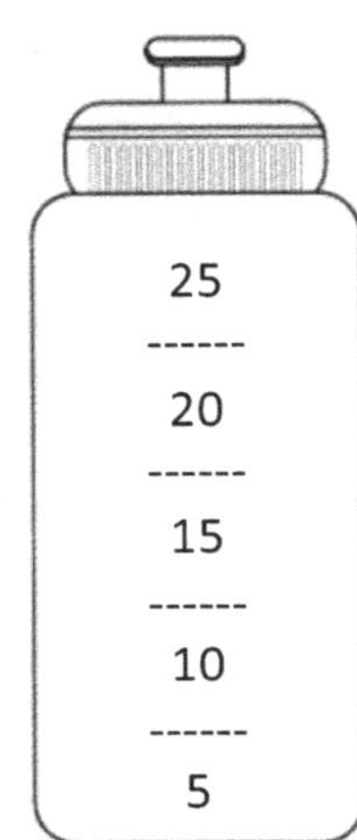 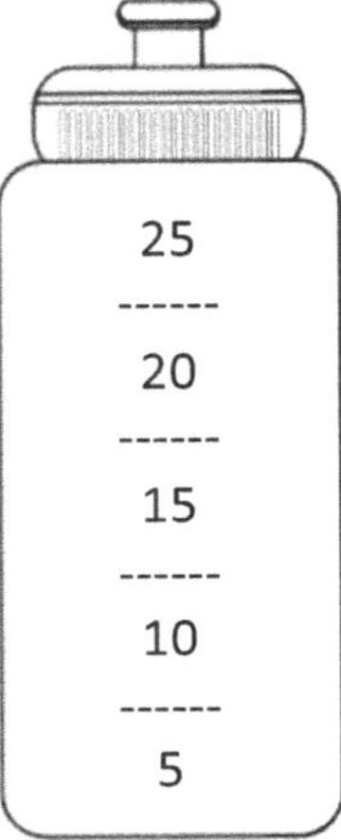

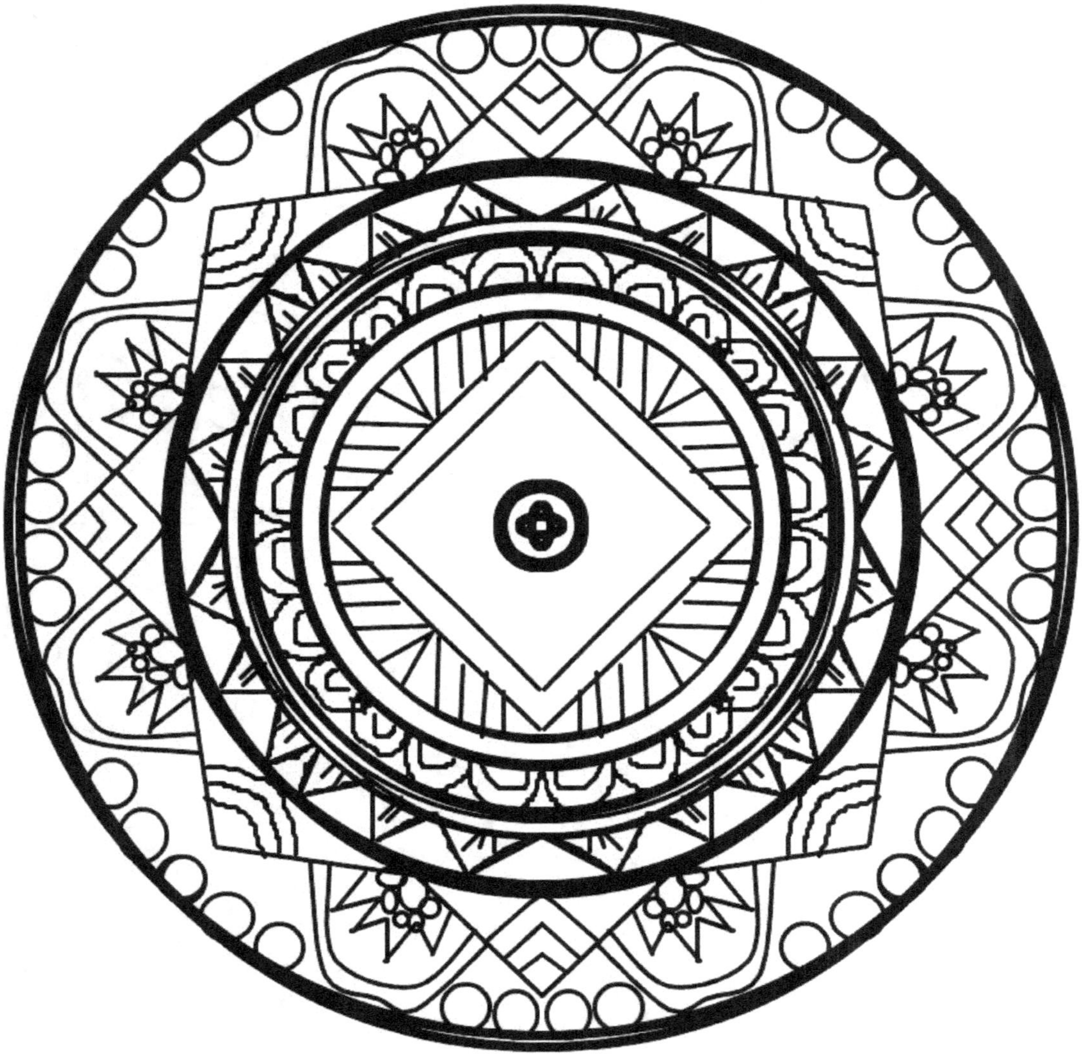

Measurements

DATE: ___________

Weight: _______

Neck _______

Shoulders _______

Chest _______

Bicep / upper arm left _________ right _______

Forearm left _________ right _______

Waist _______

Hips _______

Thighs left _________ right _______

Calf left _________ right _______

It's Not A Diet,
It's A Lifestyle Change

Day Thirty ________

5:00 ________________________

6:00 ________________________

7:00 ________________________

8:00 ________________________

9:00 ________________________

10:00 ______________________

11:00 ______________________

Noon _______________________

1:00 ________________________

2:00 ________________________

3:00 ________________________

4:00 ________________________

5:00 ________________________

6:00 ________________________

7:00 ________________________

8:00 ________________________

9:00 ________________________

10:00 ______________________

11:00 ______________________

Midnight __________________

top priorities for today

Today's victories

How can you be powerful and sensitive at the same time?

The *Stella Society* Workout

Exercise	Set 1	Set 2	Set 3	Set 4	Set 5	notes

Time started: _____________ Time ended: _____________

Location: ____

Feelings before training:

Feelings after training

NUTRITION

Meal 1

time eaten: _________

Meal 2

time eaten: _________

Meal 3

time eaten: _________

Meal 4

time eaten: _________

Meal 5

time eaten: _________

Hydration

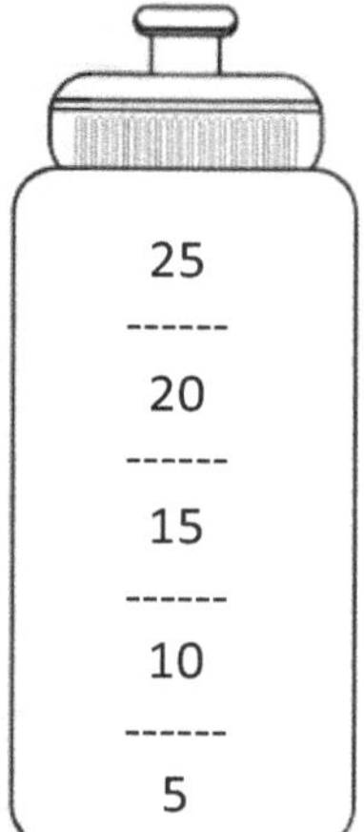

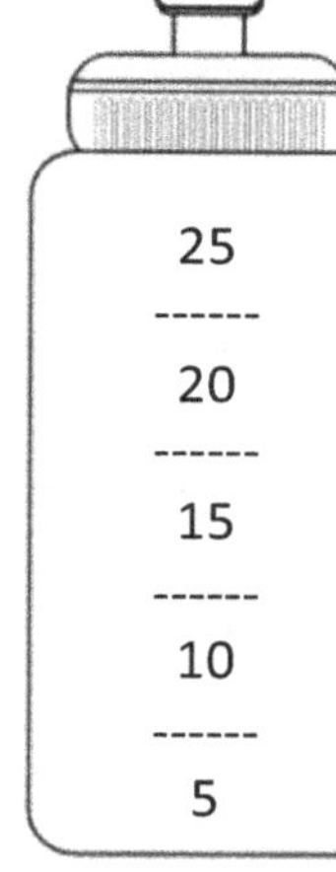

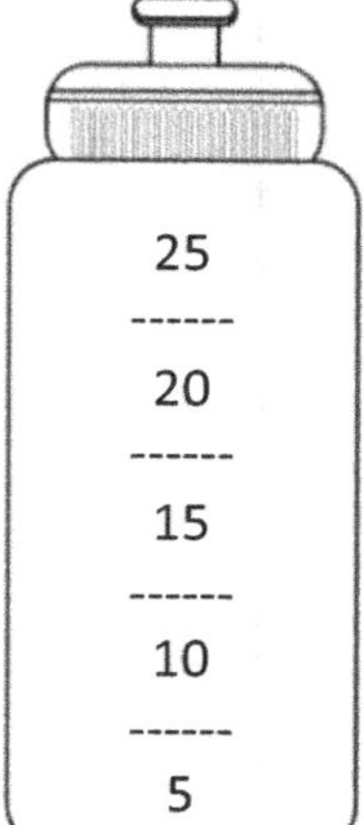

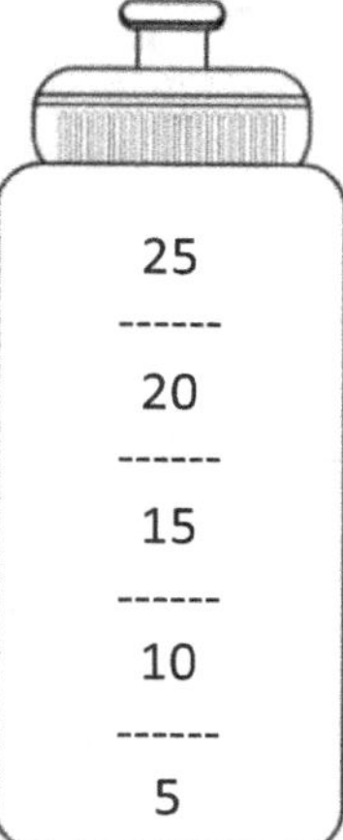

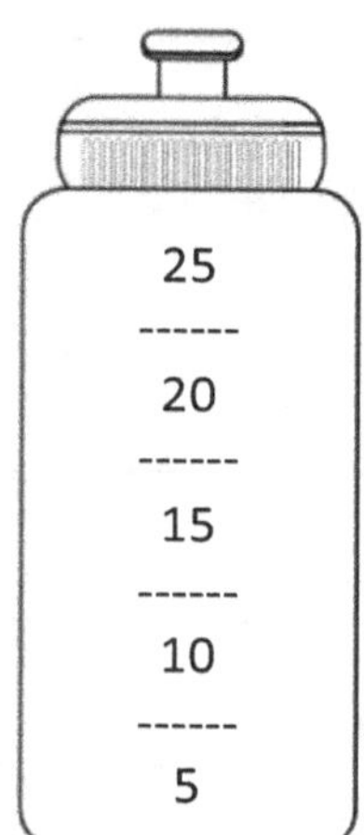

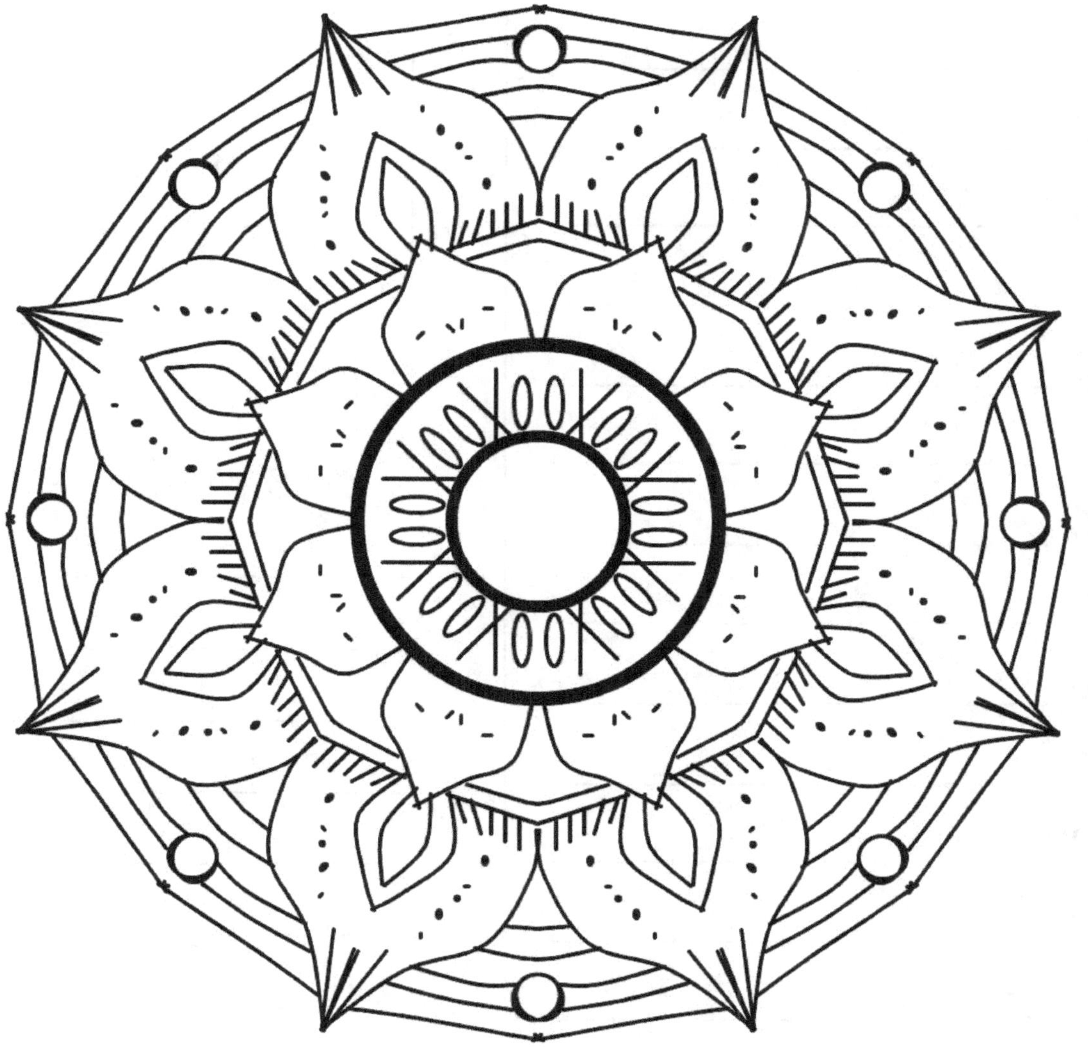

Day Thirty-one ______

5:00	______________
6:00	______________
7:00	______________
8:00	______________
9:00	______________
10:00	______________
11:00	______________
Noon	______________
1:00	______________
2:00	______________
3:00	______________
4:00	______________
5:00	______________
6:00	______________
7:00	______________
8:00	______________
9:00	______________
10:00	______________
11:00	______________
Midnight	______________

Today's victories

Is being forceful a bad thing?

The *Stella Society* Workout

Exercise	Set 1	Set 2	Set 3	Set 4	Set 5	notes

Time started: _____________ Time ended: _____________

Location: _______________________________________

Feelings before training:

Feelings after training

NUTRITION

Meal 1

time eaten: _________

Meal 2

time eaten: _________

Meal 3

time eaten: _________

Meal 4

time eaten: _________

Meal 5

time eaten: _________

Hydration

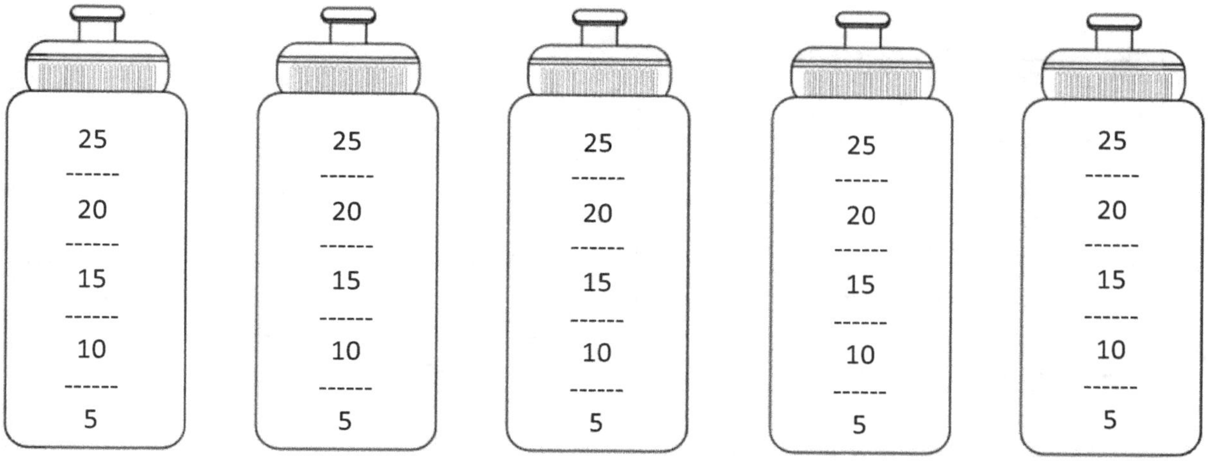

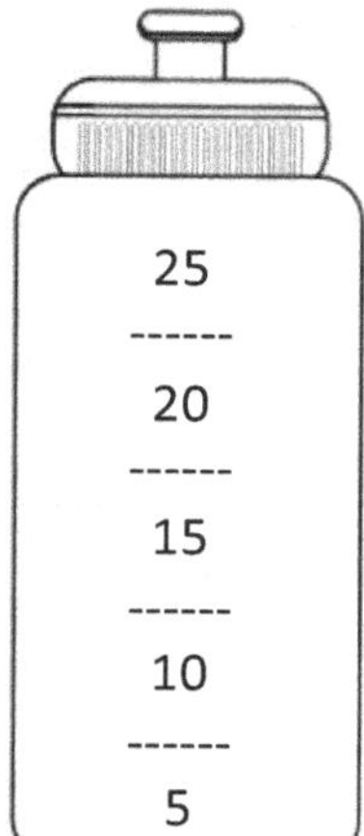 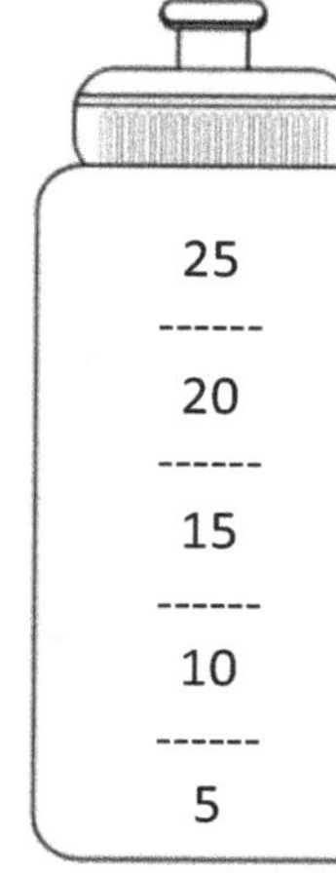

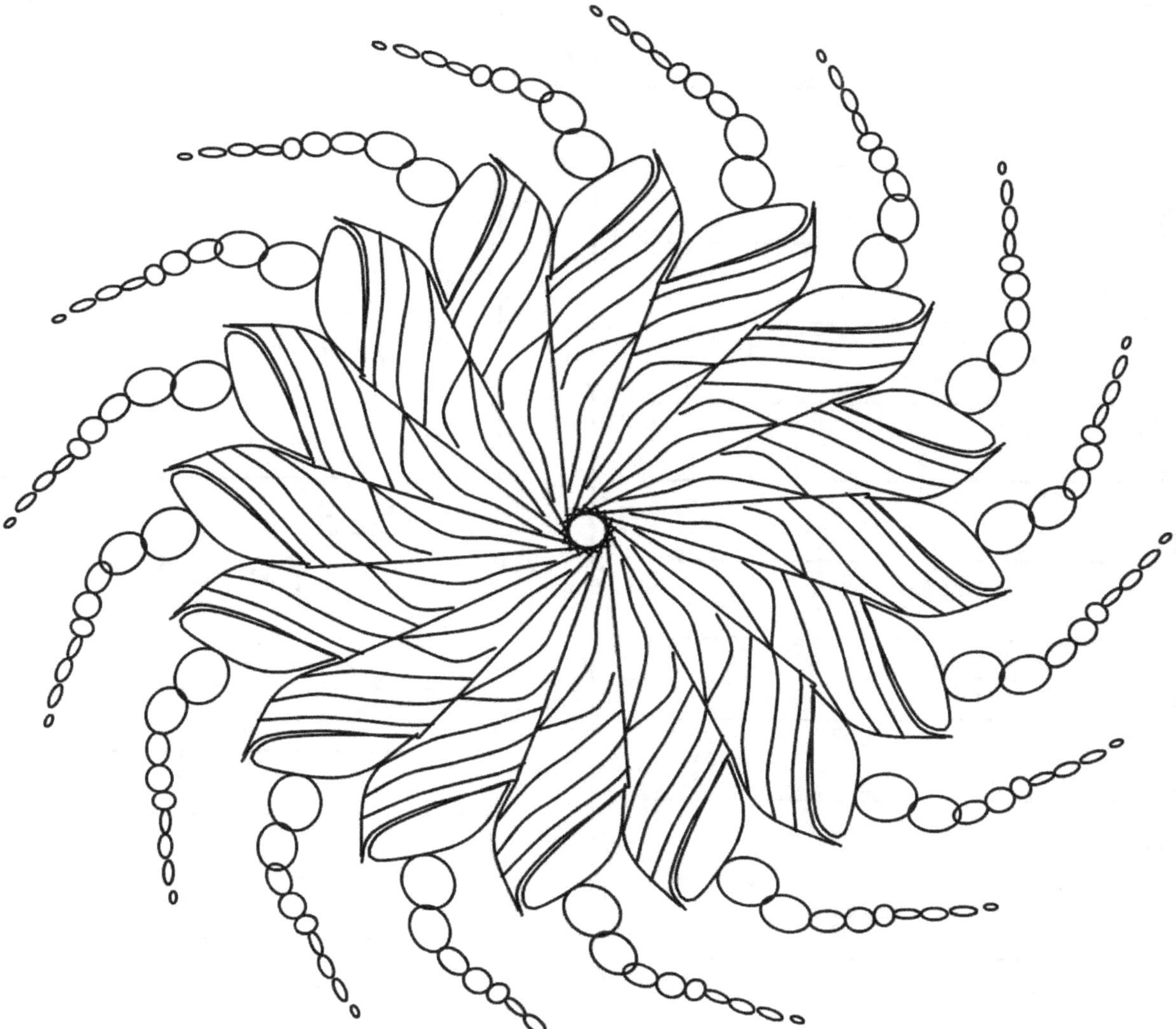

Day Thirty-two _______

<table>
<tr><td>

5:00 _______________________

6:00 _______________________

7:00 _______________________

8:00 _______________________

9:00 _______________________

10:00 ______________________

11:00 ______________________

Noon _______________________

1:00 _______________________

2:00 _______________________

3:00 _______________________

4:00 _______________________

5:00 _______________________

6:00 _______________________

7:00 _______________________

8:00 _______________________

9:00 _______________________

10:00 ______________________

11:00 ______________________

Midnight ___________________

</td><td>

top priorities for today 🎯

____

____

____

____

Today's victories 🏆

What does it mean to be fervent?

____

____

____

____

____

____

____

</td></tr>
</table>

The Stella Society Workout

Exercise	Set 1	Set 2	Set 3	Set 4	Set 5	notes

Time started: _____________   Time ended: _____________

Location: ____

Feelings before training: 🙂 😐 🙁 😜 😣 😕 😊 😎

Feelings after training 🙂 😐 🙁 😜 😣 😕 😊 😎

NUTRITION

Meal 1
time eaten: _________

Meal 2
time eaten: _________

Meal 3
time eaten: _________

Meal 4
time eaten: _________

Meal 5
time eaten: _________

Hydration

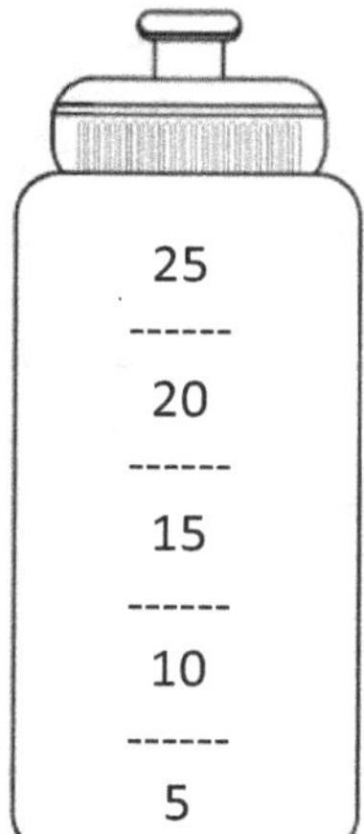

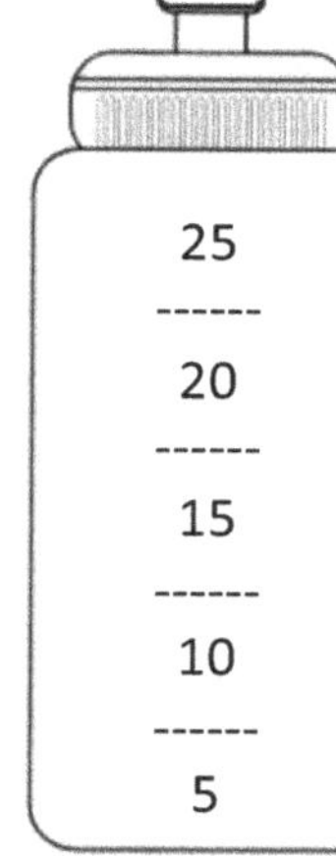

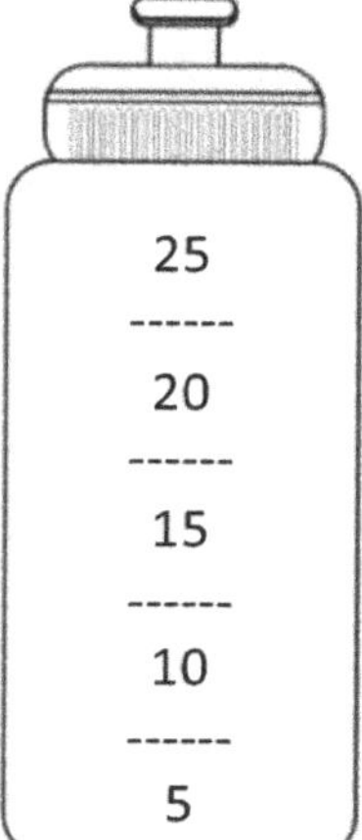

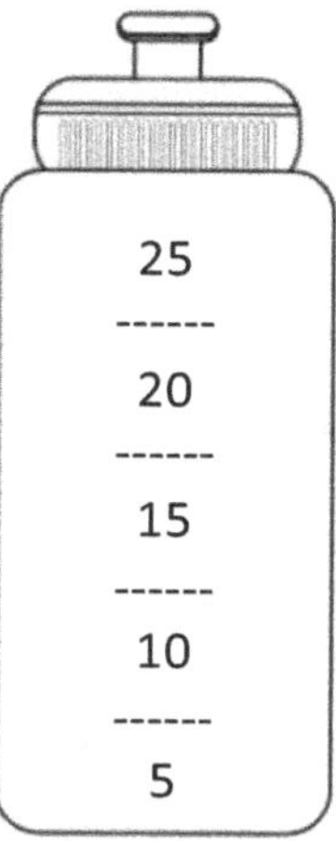

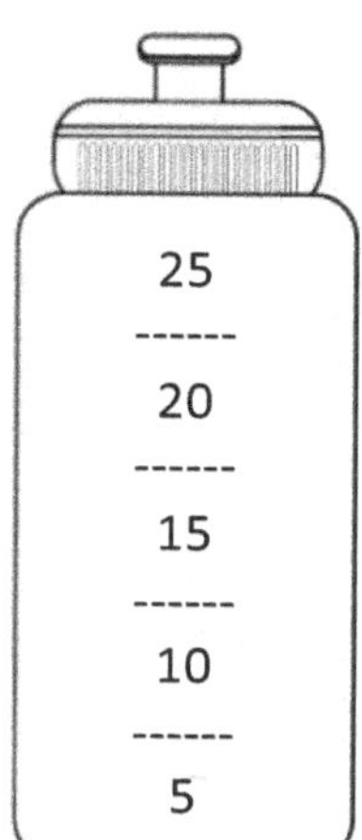

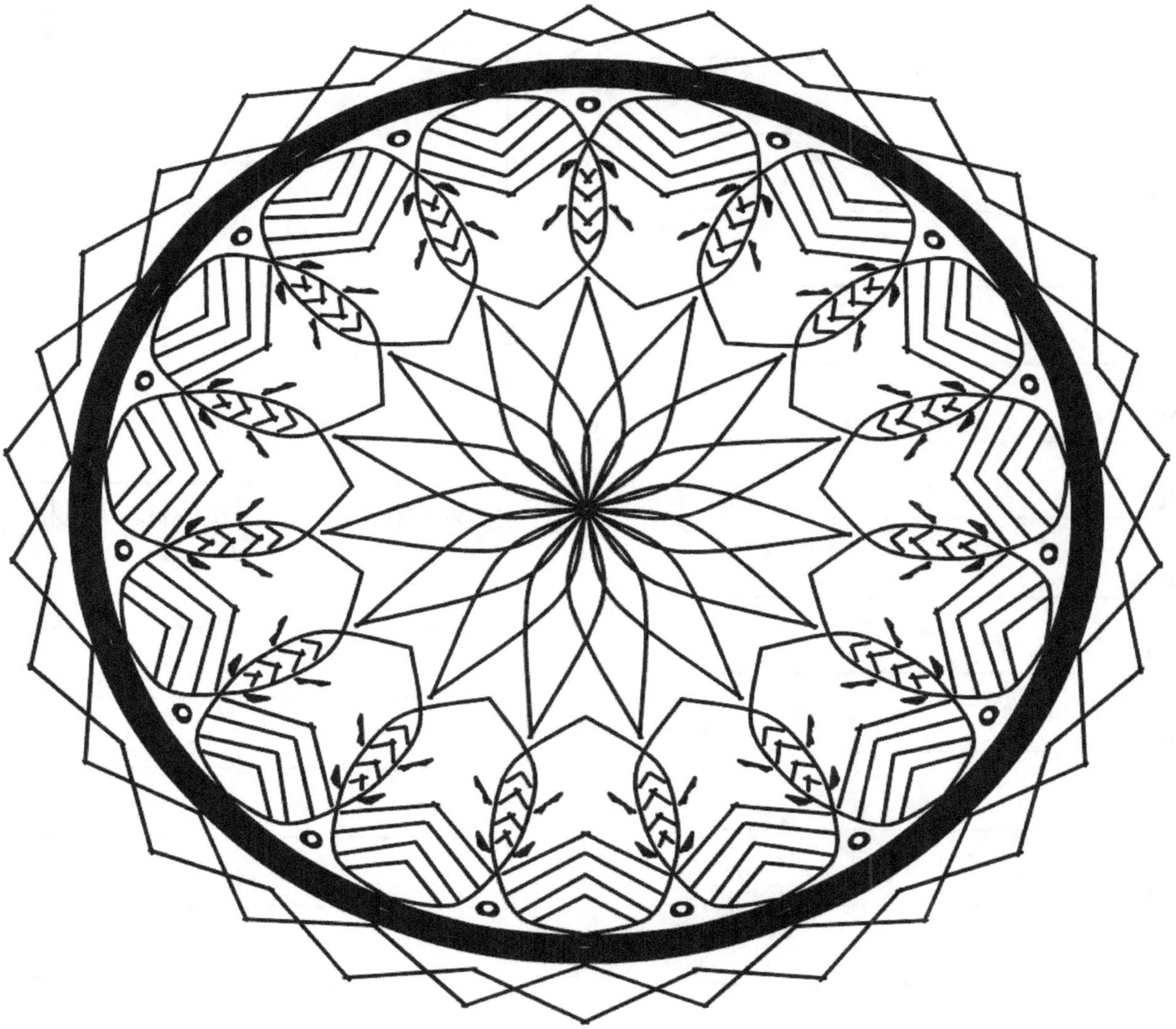

Day Thirty-three _______

5:00 _______________________

6:00 _______________________

7:00 _______________________

8:00 _______________________

9:00 _______________________

10:00 ______________________

11:00 ______________________

Noon _______________________

1:00 _______________________

2:00 _______________________

3:00 _______________________

4:00 _______________________

5:00 _______________________

6:00 _______________________

7:00 _______________________

8:00 _______________________

9:00 _______________________

10:00 ______________________

11:00 ______________________

Midnight ____________________

____

____

____

____

How are you glowing today?

____

____

____

____

____

____

The *Stella Society* Workout

Exercise	Set 1	Set 2	Set 3	Set 4	Set 5	notes

Time started: _____________   Time ended: _______________

Location: ____

Feelings before training: 🙂 😐 🙁 😜 😣 🙁 😊 😎

Feelings after training 🙂 😐 🙁 😜 😣 🙁 😊 😎

NUTRITION

Meal 1

time eaten: _________

Meal 2

time eaten: _________

Meal 3

time eaten: _________

Meal 4

time eaten: _________

Meal 5

time eaten: _________

Hydration

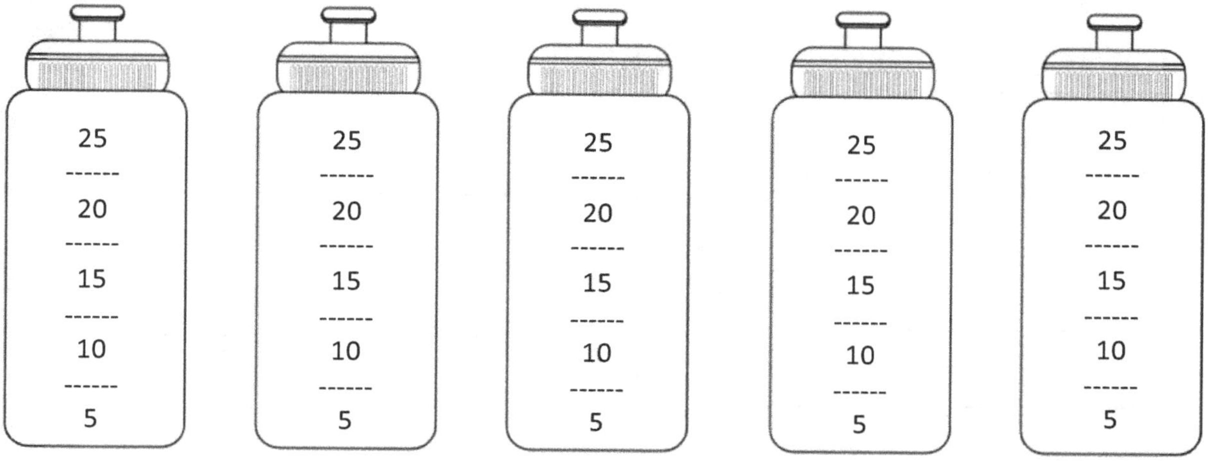

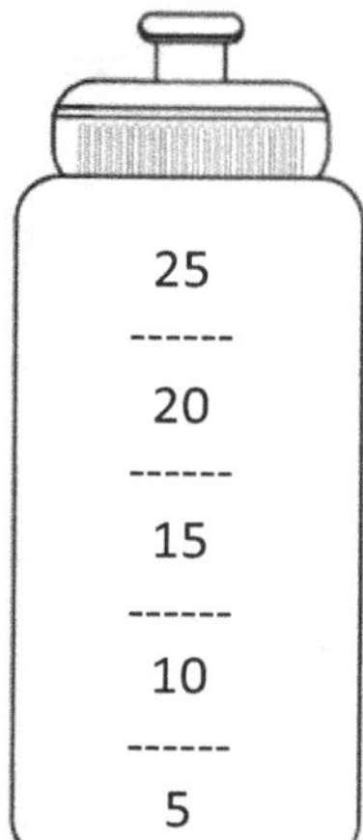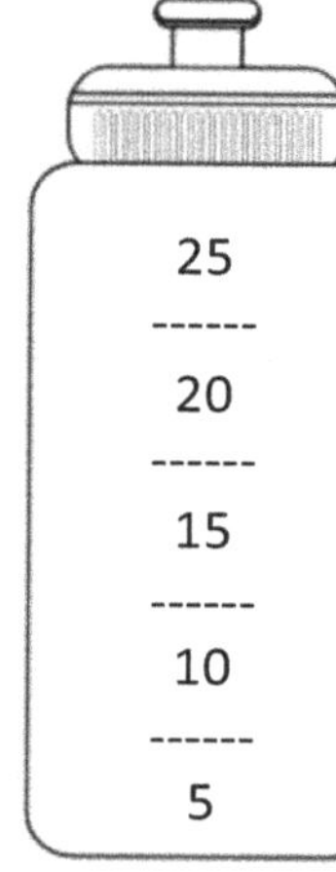

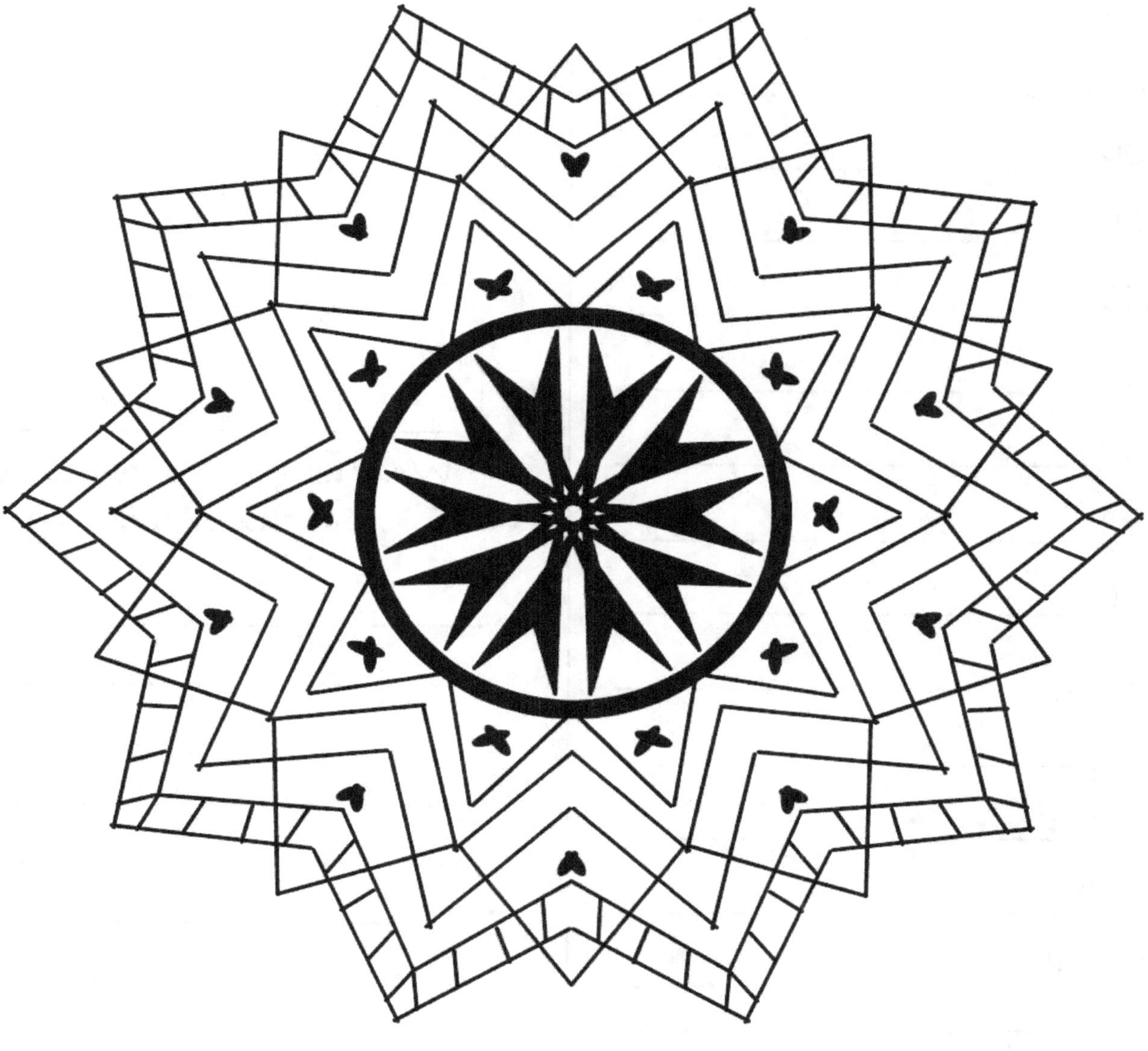

Day Thirty-four _______

5:00 _______________________

6:00 _______________________

7:00 _______________________

8:00 _______________________

9:00 _______________________

10:00 _______________________

11:00 _______________________

Noon _______________________

1:00 _______________________

2:00 _______________________

3:00 _______________________

4:00 _______________________

5:00 _______________________

6:00 _______________________

7:00 _______________________

8:00 _______________________

9:00 _______________________

10:00 _______________________

11:00 _______________________

Midnight _______________________

Today's victories

What are you dedicated to
do at this moment?

The Stella Society Workout

Exercise	Set 1	Set 2	Set 3	Set 4	Set 5	notes

Time started: _____________   Time ended: _____________

Location: ____

Feelings before training: 😊 😐 ☹️ 😜 😠 😕 😊 😎

Feelings after training 😊 😐 ☹️ 😜 😠 😕 😊 😎

NUTRITION

Meal 1

time eaten: _________

Meal 2

time eaten: _________

Meal 3

time eaten: _________

Meal 4

time eaten: _________

Meal 5

time eaten: _________

Hydration

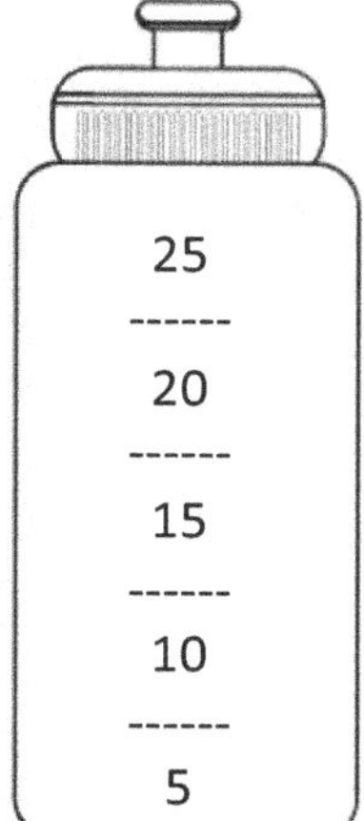

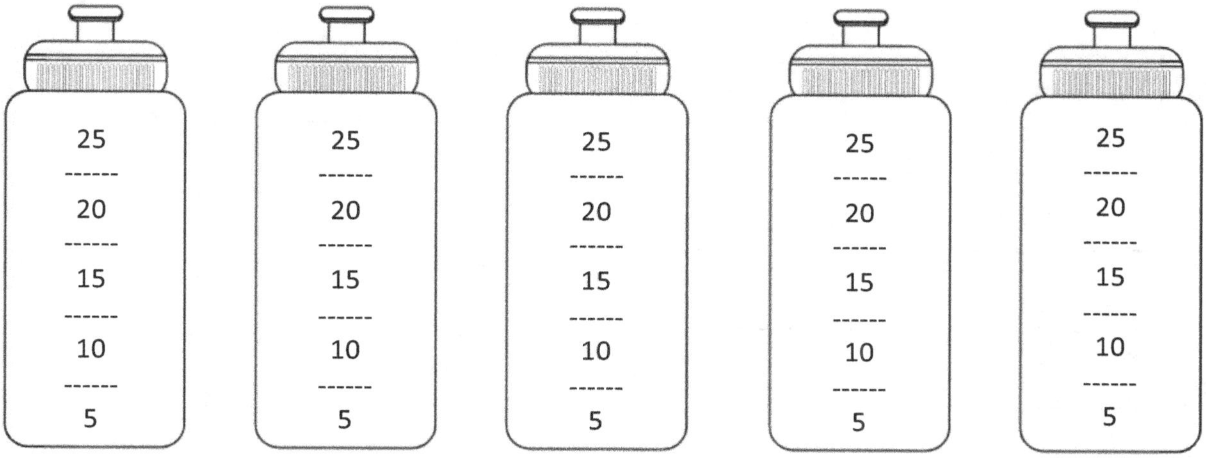

25

20

15

10

5

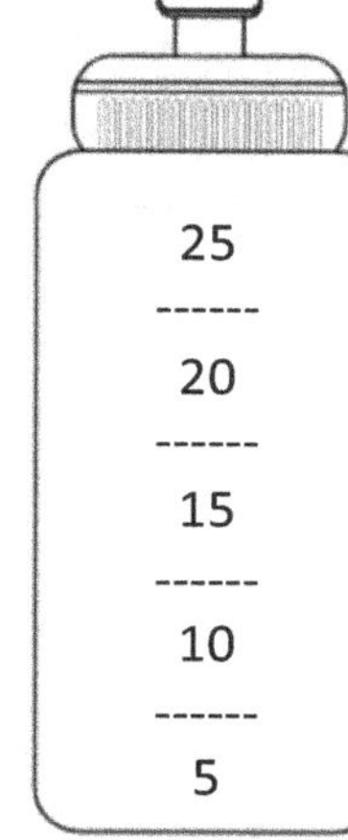

25

20

15

10

5

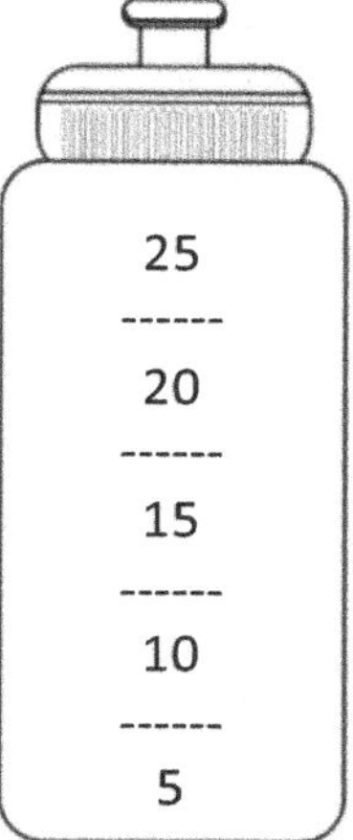

25

20

15

10

5

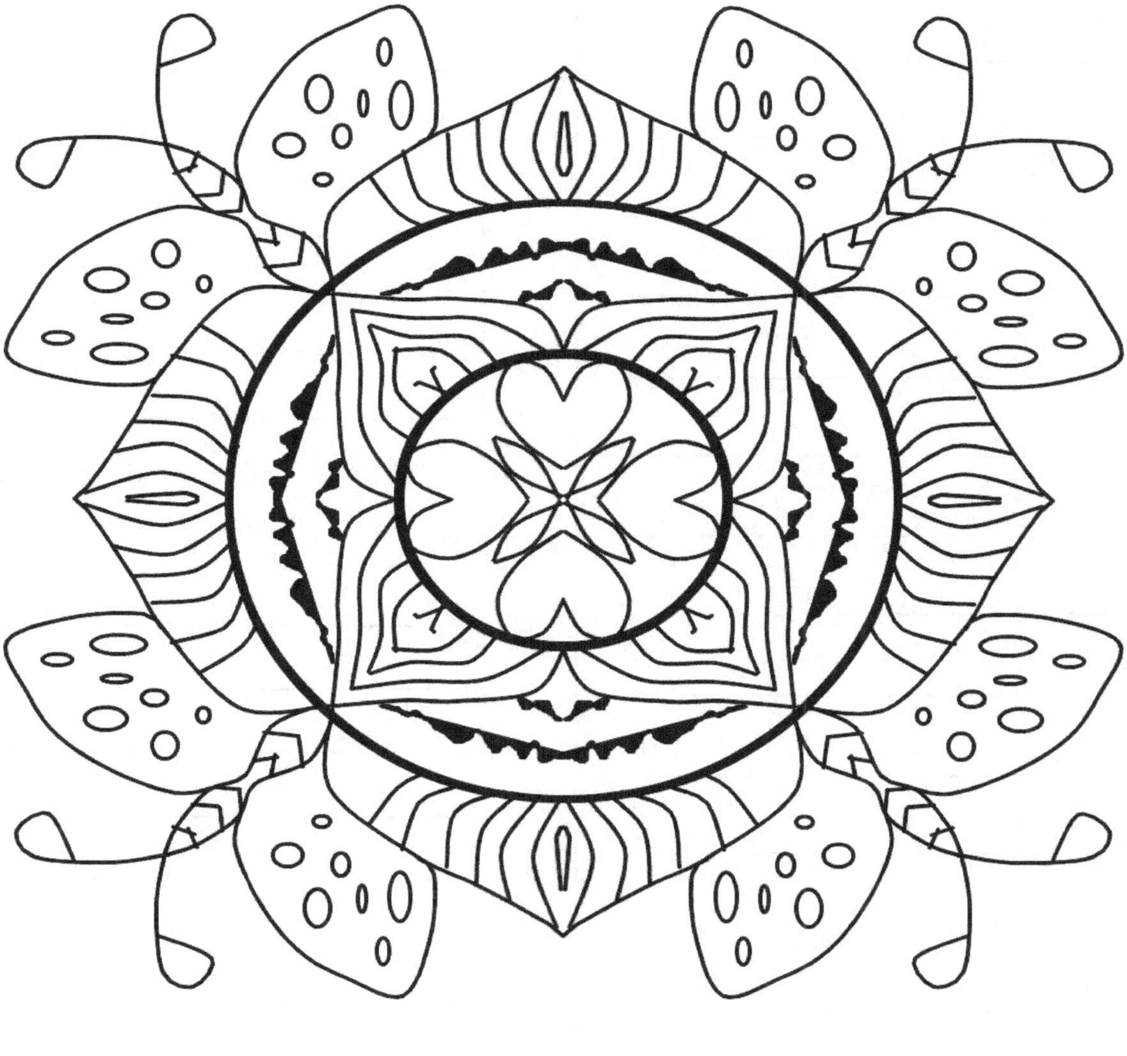

Day Thirty-five _______

5:00 _______________________

6:00 _______________________

7:00 _______________________

8:00 _______________________

9:00 _______________________

10:00 ______________________

11:00 ______________________

Noon _______________________

1:00 _______________________

2:00 _______________________

3:00 _______________________

4:00 _______________________

5:00 _______________________

6:00 _______________________

7:00 _______________________

8:00 _______________________

9:00 _______________________

10:00 ______________________

11:00 ______________________

Midnight ___________________

____

____

____

____

Today's victories

Who is more determined
than you?

____

____

____

____

____

____

The Stella Society Workout

Exercise	Set 1	Set 2	Set 3	Set 4	Set 5	notes

Time started: _____________ Time ended: _____________

Location: ____

Feelings before training: 🙂 😐 🙁 😜 😠 😕 😊 😎

Feelings after training 🙂 😐 🙁 😜 😠 😕 😊 😎

NUTRITION

Meal 1
time eaten: _________

Meal 2
time eaten: _________

Meal 3
time eaten: _________

Meal 4
time eaten: _________

Meal 5
time eaten: _________

Hydration

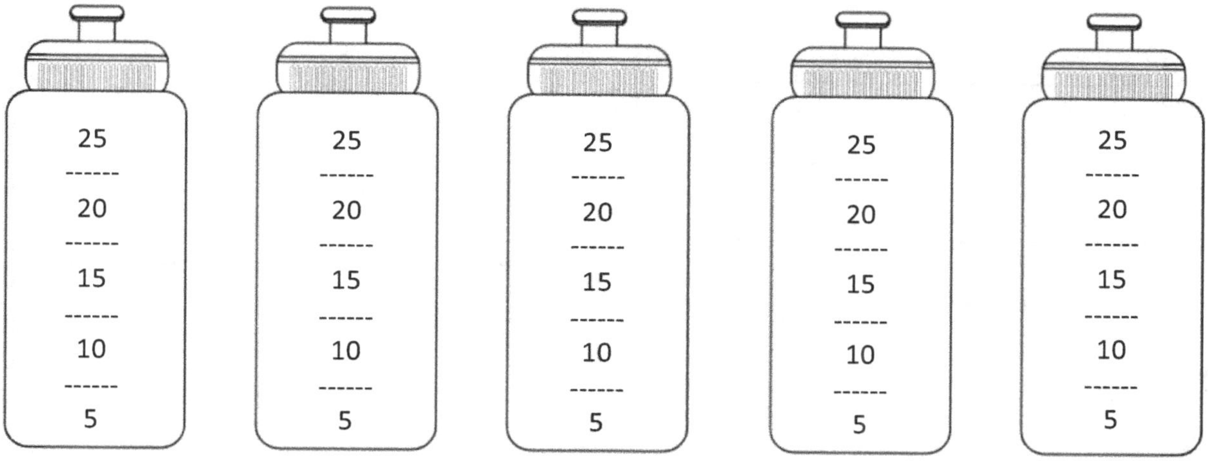

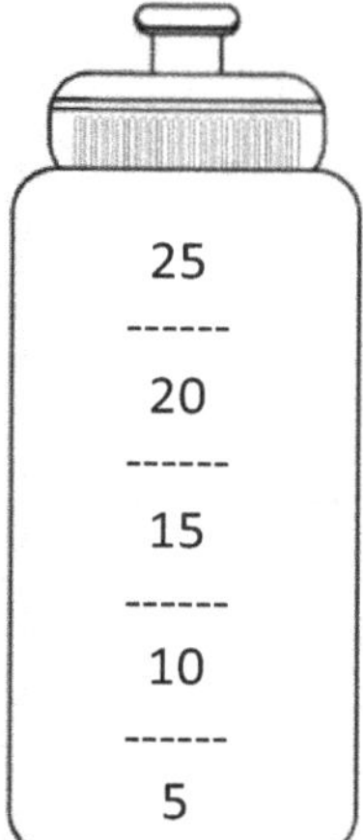

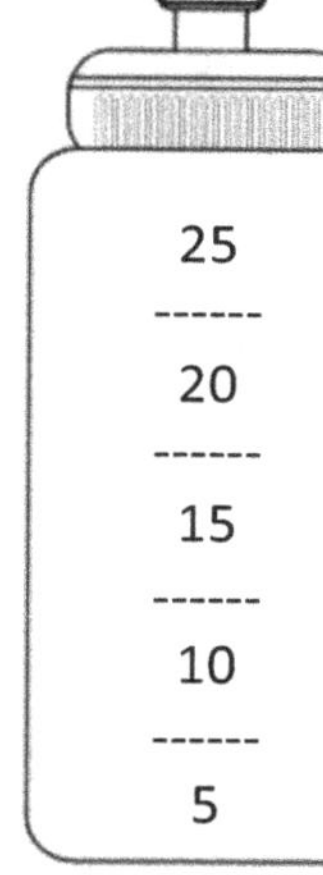

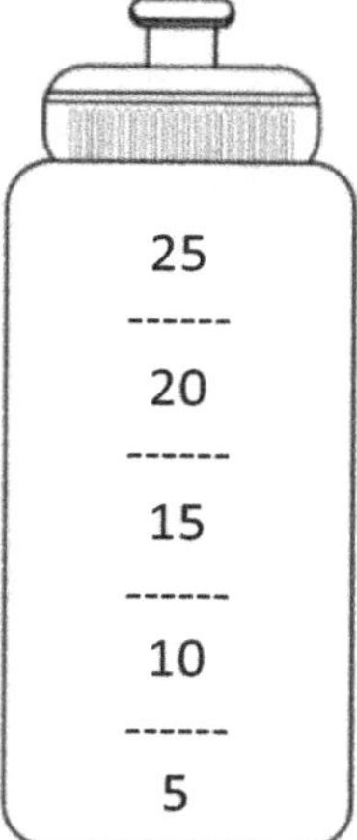

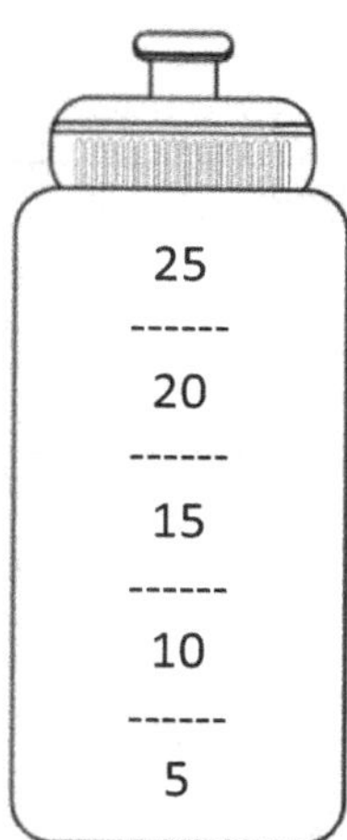

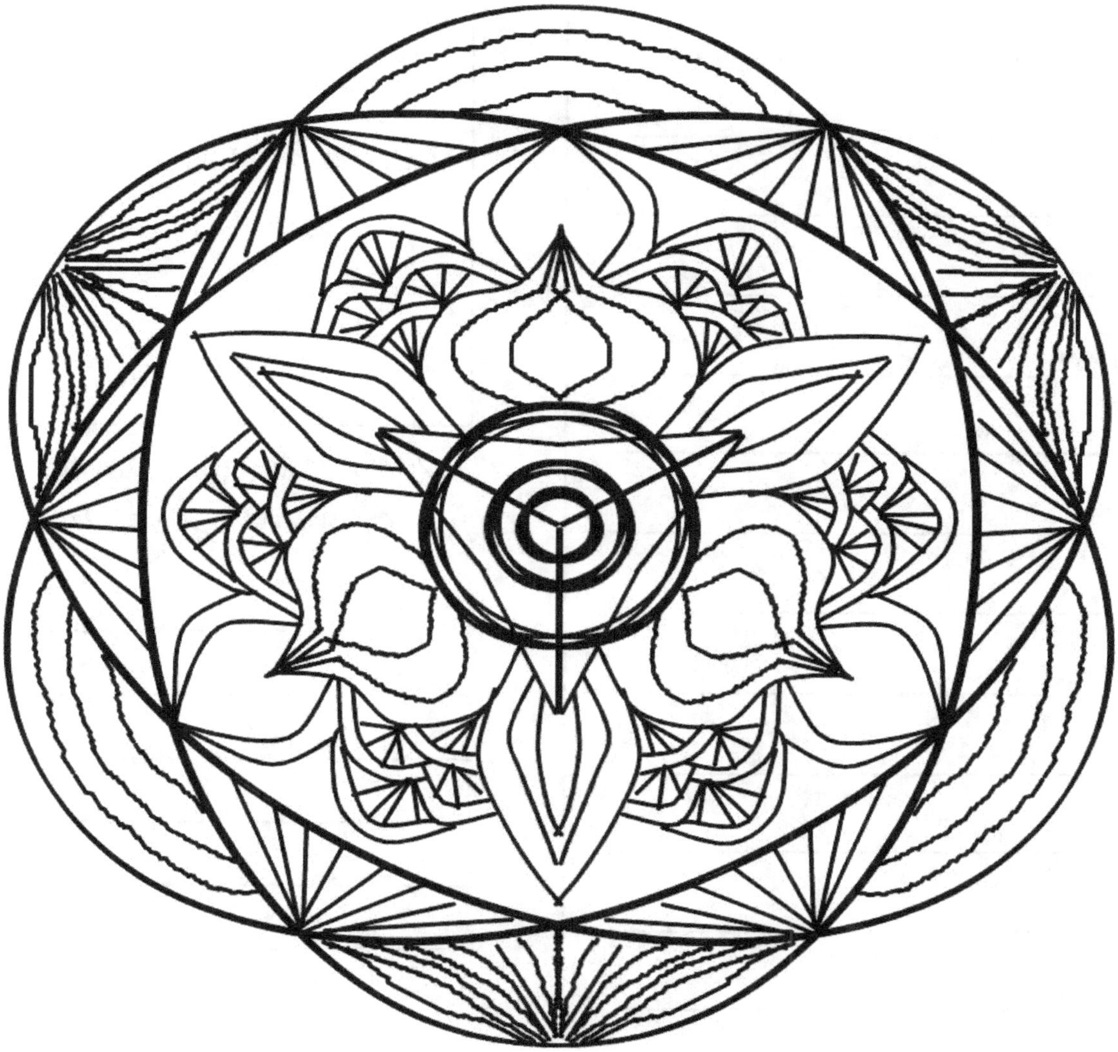

Day Thirty-six _______

top priorities for today

5:00	
6:00	
7:00	
8:00	
9:00	
10:00	
11:00	
Noon	
1:00	
2:00	
3:00	
4:00	
5:00	
6:00	
7:00	
8:00	
9:00	
10:00	
11:00	
Midnight	

Today's victories

Who needs your acceptance of change and why?

The *Stella Society* Workout

Exercise	Set 1	Set 2	Set 3	Set 4	Set 5	notes

Time started: _____________ Time ended: _____________

Location: ____

Feelings before training: ☺ 😐 ☹ 😜 😠 😕 😇 😎

Feelings after training ☺ 😐 ☹ 😜 😠 😕 😇 😎

NUTRITION

Meal 1

time eaten: _________

Meal 2

time eaten: _________

Meal 3

time eaten: _________

Meal 4

time eaten: _________

Meal 5

time eaten: _________

Hydration

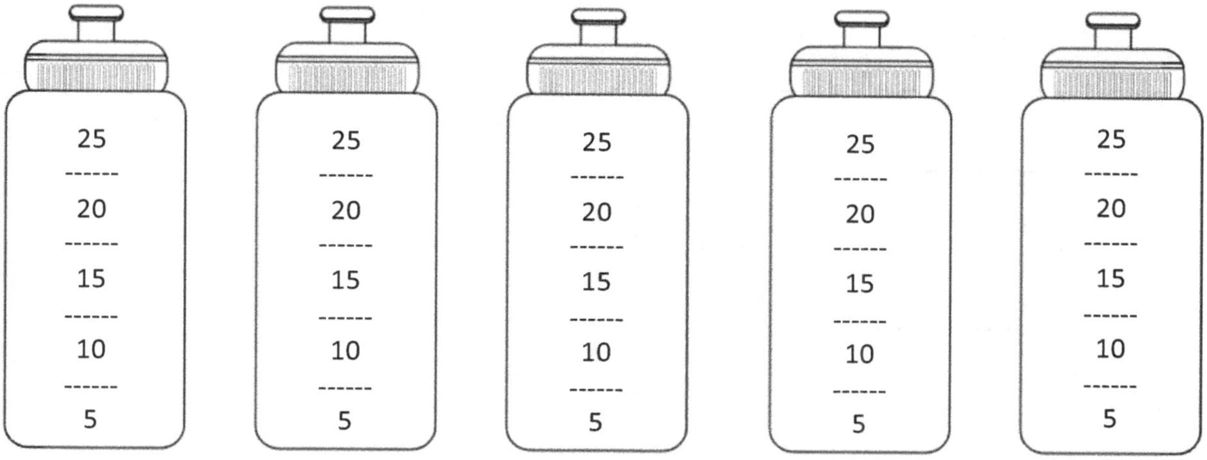

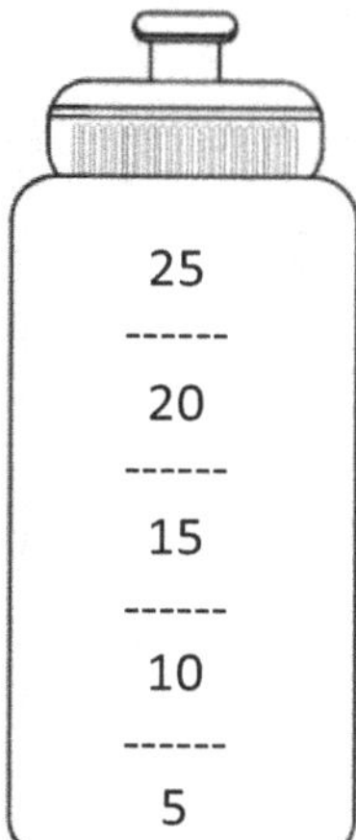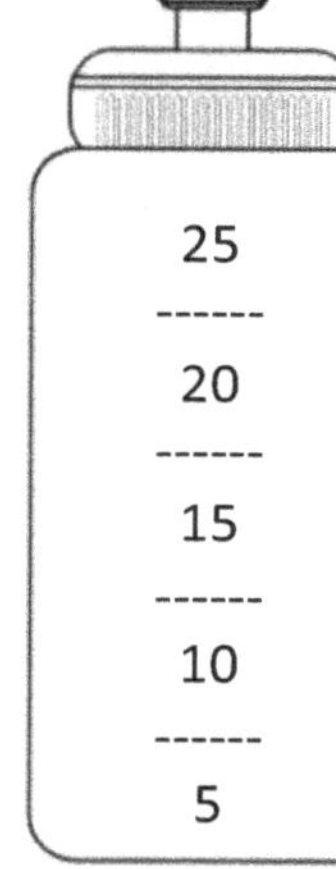

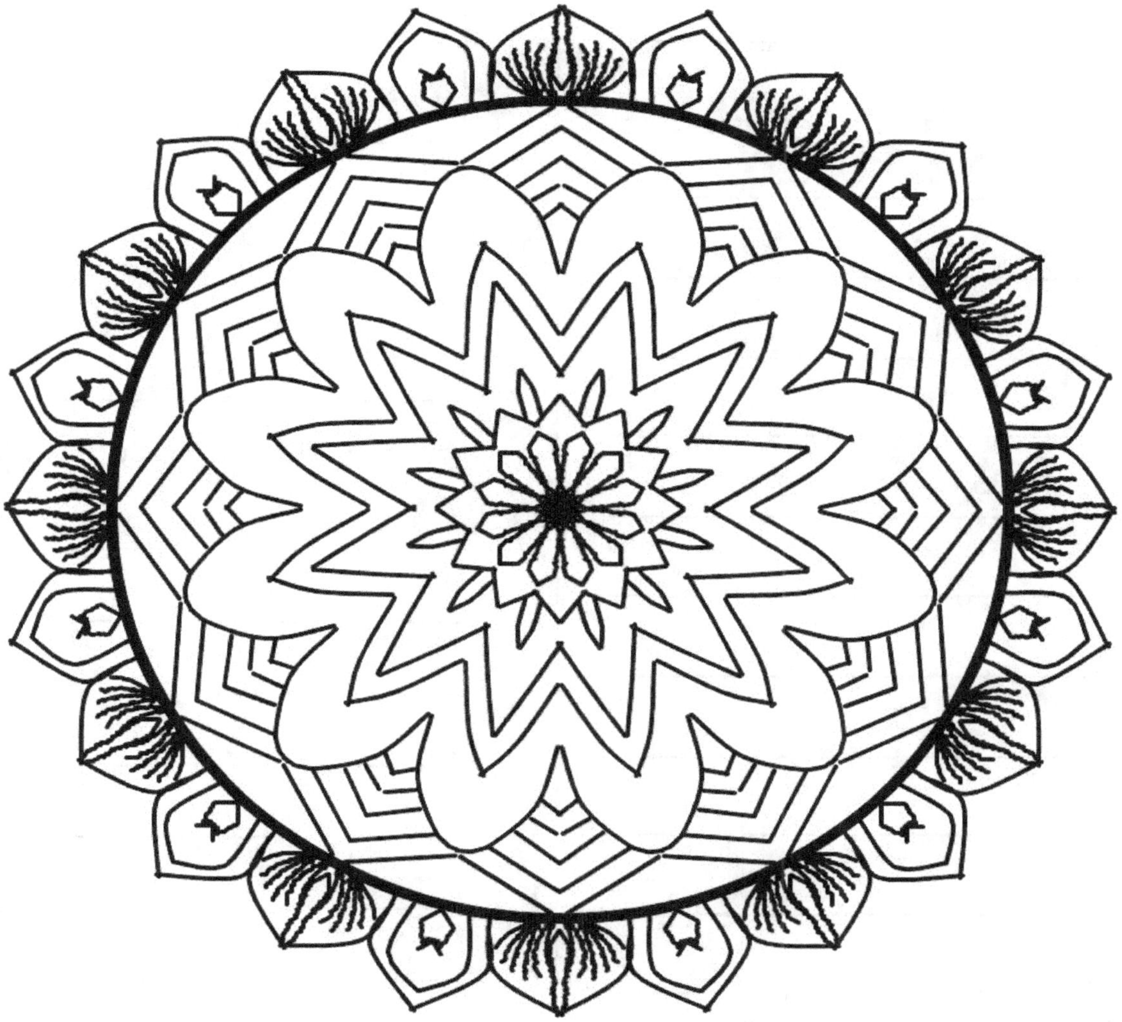

Day Thirty-seven _______

5:00 _______________________

6:00 _______________________

7:00 _______________________

8:00 _______________________

9:00 _______________________

10:00 _______________________

11:00 _______________________

Noon _______________________

1:00 _______________________

2:00 _______________________

3:00 _______________________

4:00 _______________________

5:00 _______________________

6:00 _______________________

7:00 _______________________

8:00 _______________________

9:00 _______________________

10:00 _______________________

11:00 _______________________

Midnight _______________________

top priorities for today 🎯

____

____

____

____

____

Today's victories 🏆

How will you be captivating?

____

____

____

____

____

____

The *Stella Society* Workout

Exercise	Set 1	Set 2	Set 3	Set 4	Set 5	notes

Time started: ________________ Time ended: ________________

Location: ____

Feelings before training: 🙂 😐 🙁 😜 😠 😕 😊 😎

Feelings after training 🙂 😐 🙁 😜 😠 😕 😊 😎

NUTRITION

Meal 1

time eaten: _________

Meal 2

time eaten: _________

Meal 3

time eaten: _________

Meal 4

time eaten: _________

Meal 5

time eaten: _________

Hydration

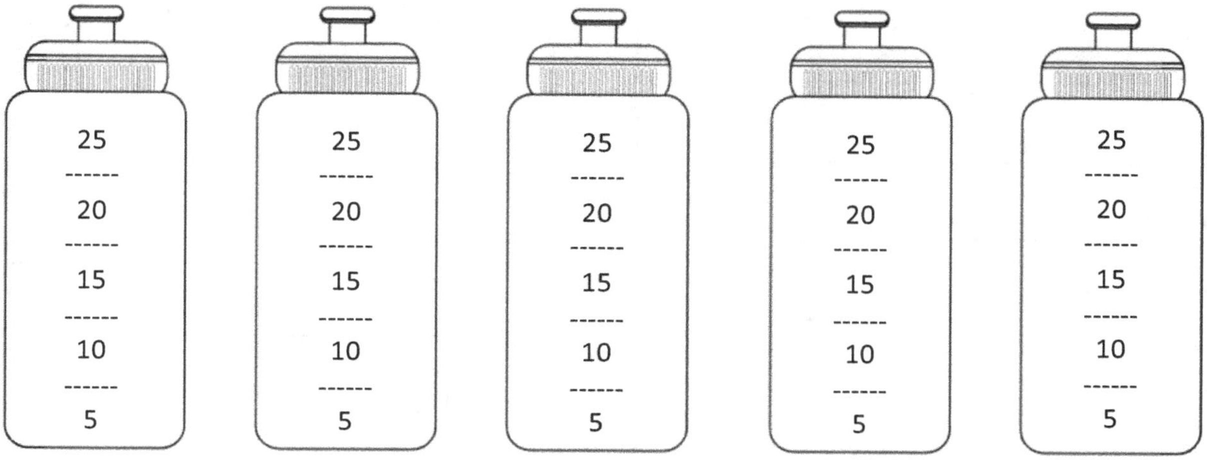

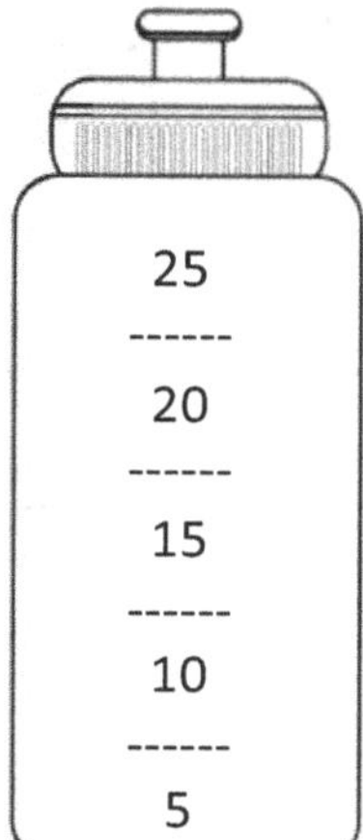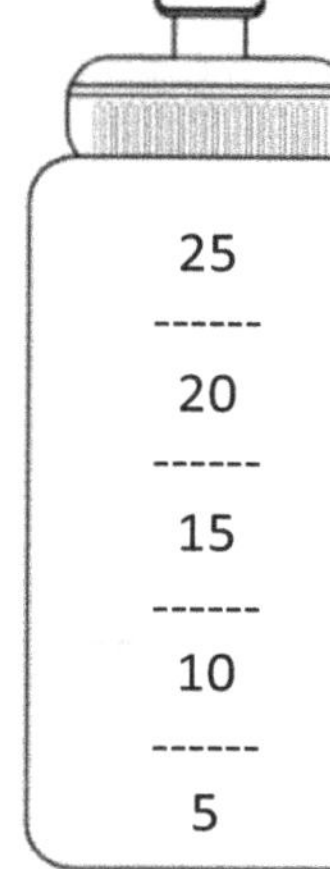

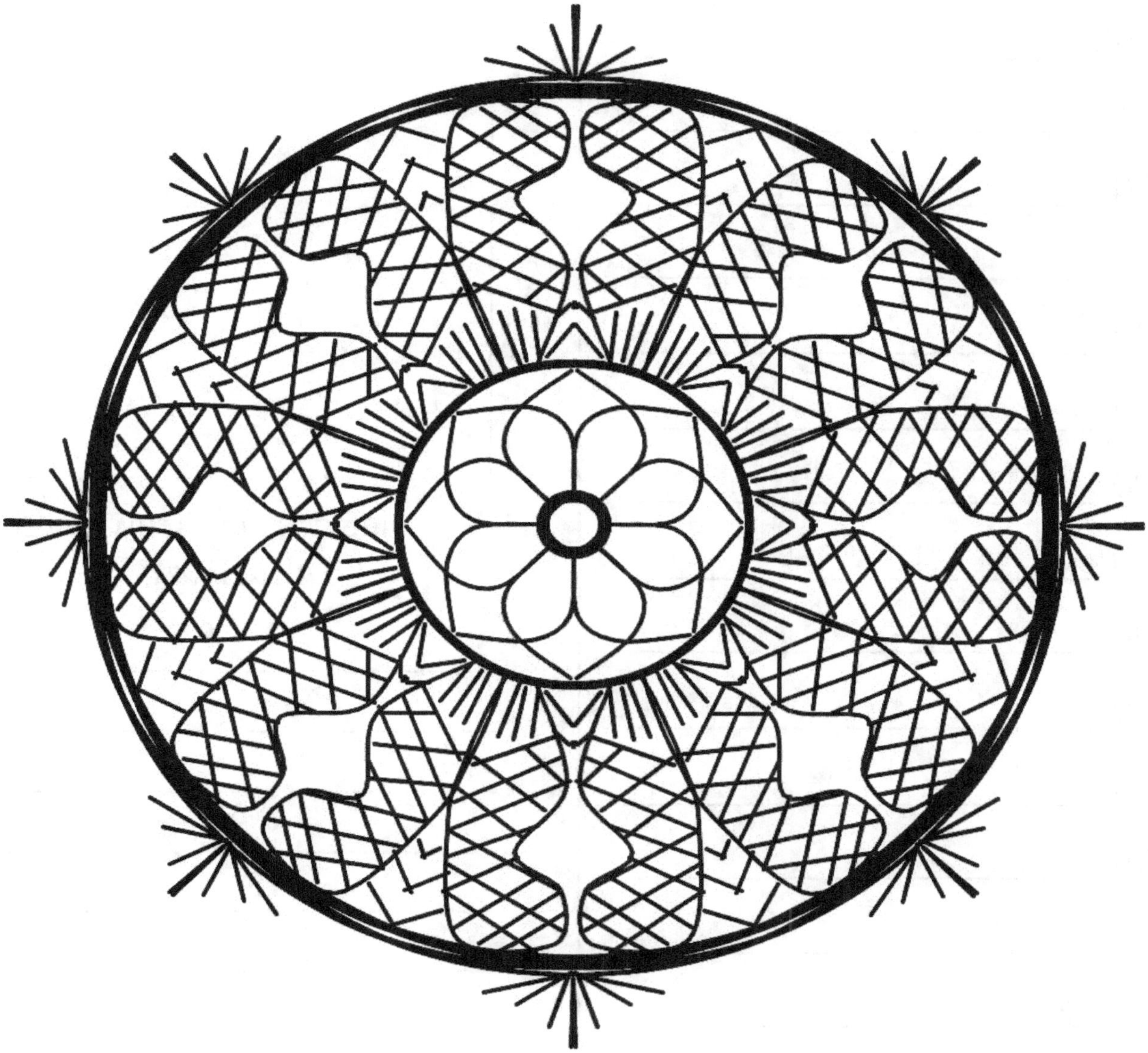

Day Thirty-eight _______

5:00 _______________________

6:00 _______________________

7:00 _______________________

8:00 _______________________

9:00 _______________________

10:00 ______________________

11:00 ______________________

Noon _______________________

1:00 _______________________

2:00 _______________________

3:00 _______________________

4:00 _______________________

5:00 _______________________

6:00 _______________________

7:00 _______________________

8:00 _______________________

9:00 _______________________

10:00 ______________________

11:00 ______________________

Midnight ____________________

top priorities for today 

____

____

____

____

Today's victories

What does it mean to be alluring?

____

____

____

____

____

____

The Stella Society Workout

Exercise	Set 1	Set 2	Set 3	Set 4	Set 5	notes

Time started: ______________   Time ended: ______________

Location: ____

Feelings before training:

Feelings after training

NUTRITION

Meal 1

time eaten: _________

Meal 2

time eaten: _________

Meal 3

time eaten: _________

Meal 4

time eaten: _________

Meal 5

time eaten: _________

Hydration

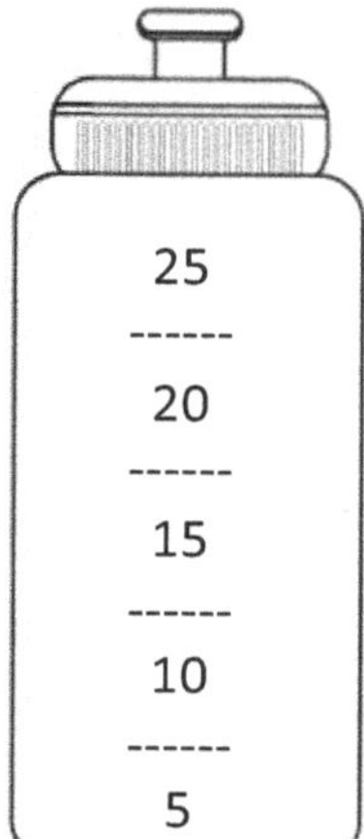

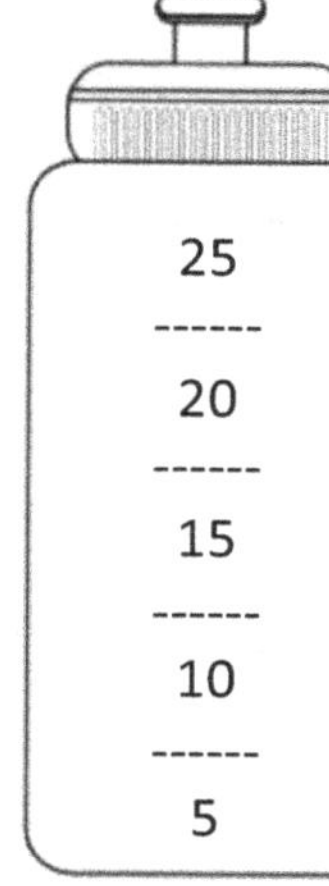

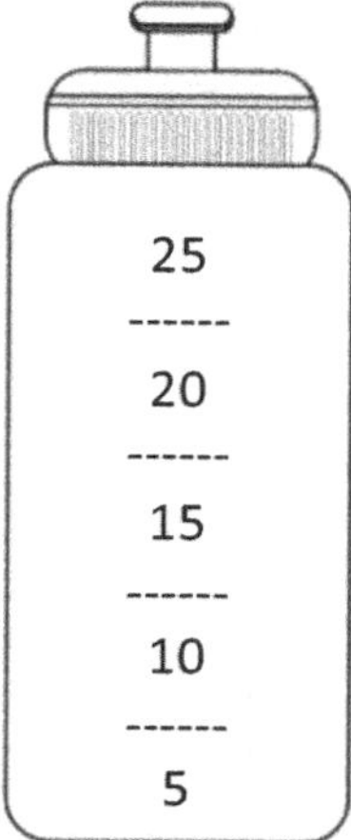

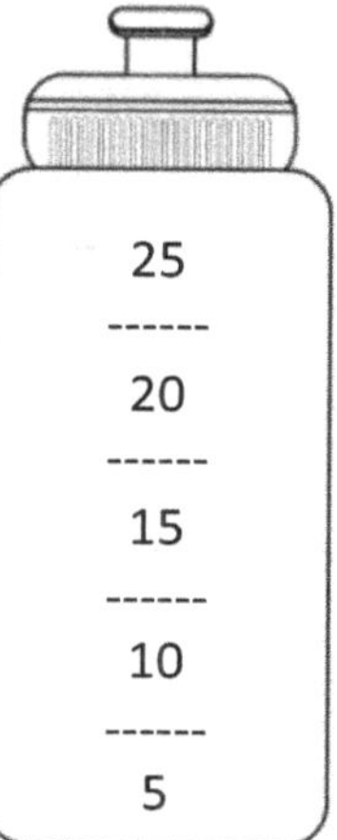

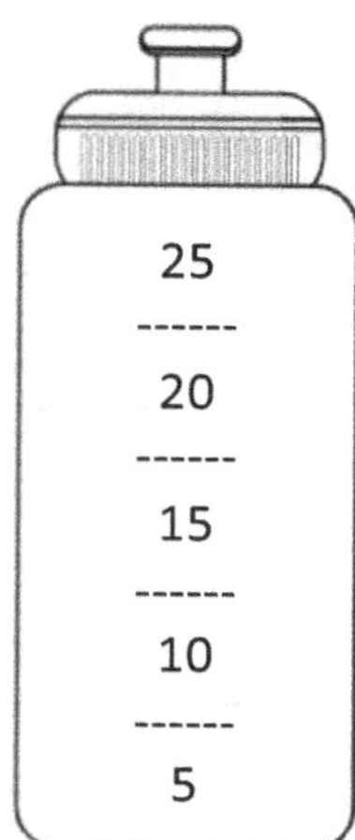

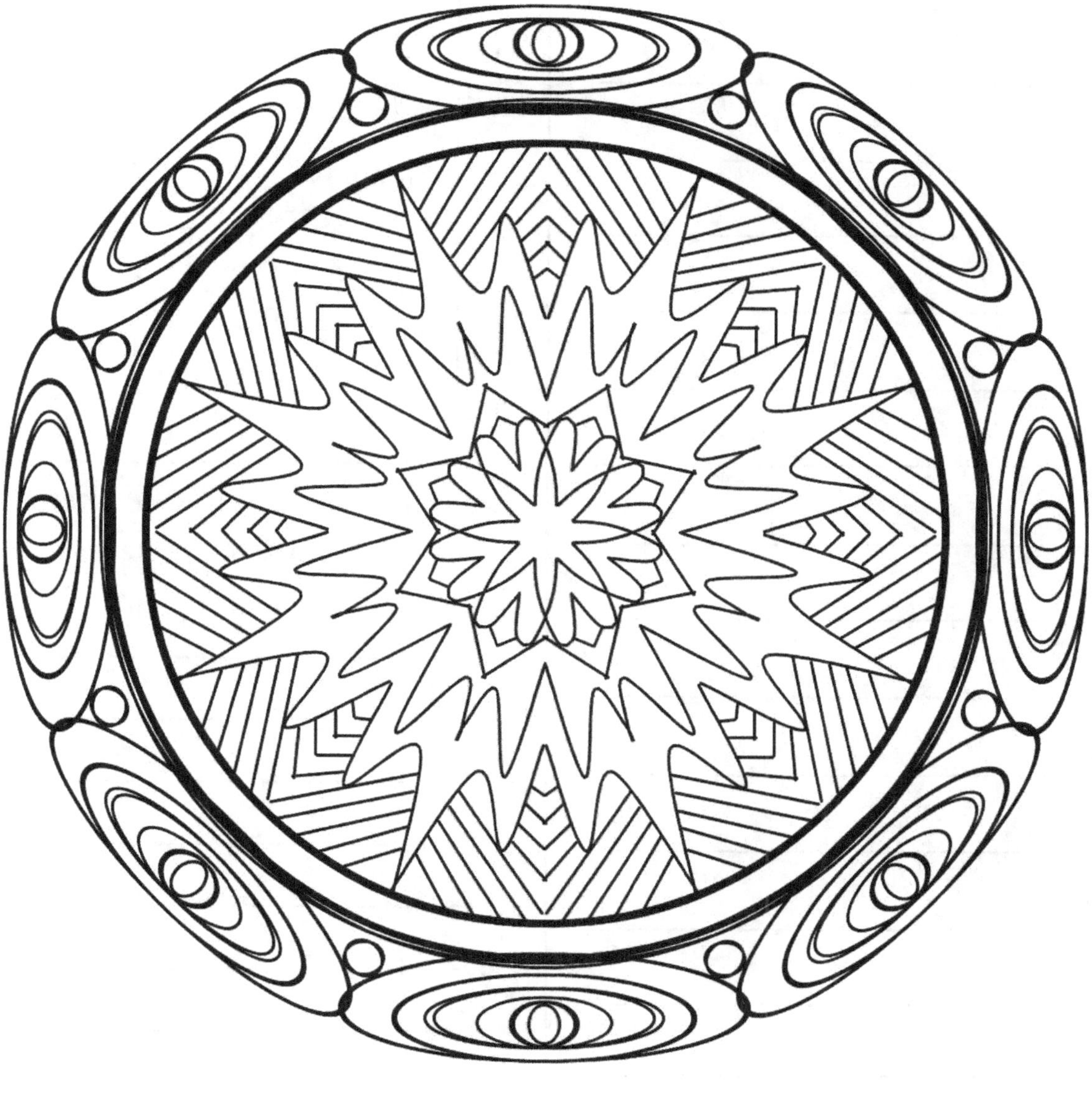

Day Thirty-nine ______

5:00 ________________	

5:00 ______________________
6:00 ______________________
7:00 ______________________
8:00 ______________________
9:00 ______________________
10:00 _____________________
11:00 _____________________
Noon ______________________
1:00 ______________________
2:00 ______________________
3:00 ______________________
4:00 ______________________
5:00 ______________________
6:00 ______________________
7:00 ______________________
8:00 ______________________
9:00 ______________________
10:00 _____________________
11:00 _____________________
Midnight ___________________

____
____
____
____

How will you be the best
version of you?

____
____
____
____
____
____

The Stella Society Workout

Exercise	Set 1	Set 2	Set 3	Set 4	Set 5	notes

Time started: ______________   Time ended: ______________

Location: ____

Feelings before training:

Feelings after training

NUTRITION

Meal 1
time eaten: _________

Meal 2
time eaten: _________

Meal 3
time eaten: _________

Meal 4
time eaten: _________

Meal 5
time eaten: _________

Hydration

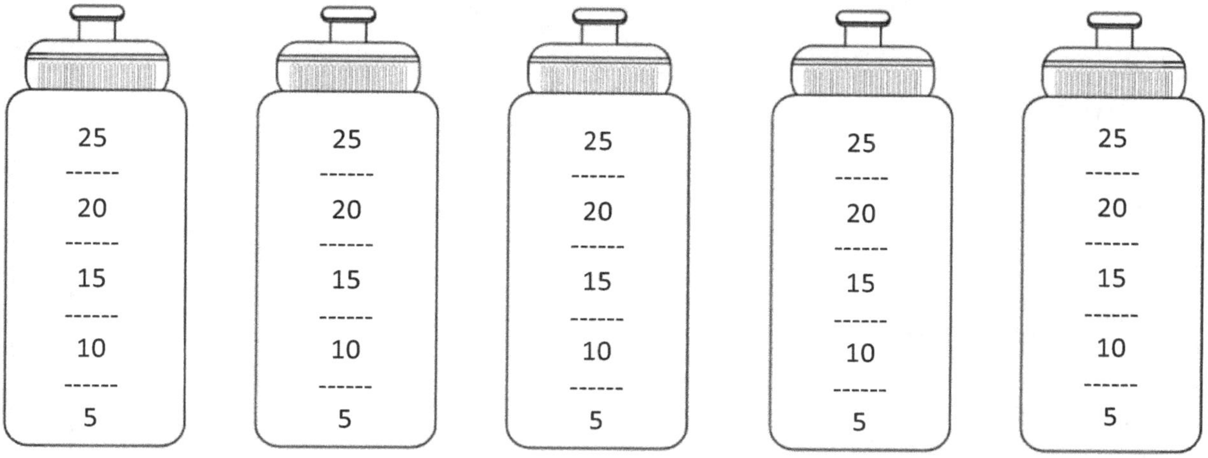

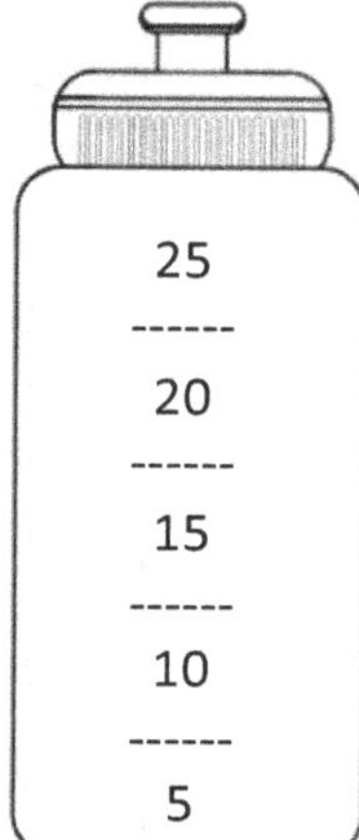
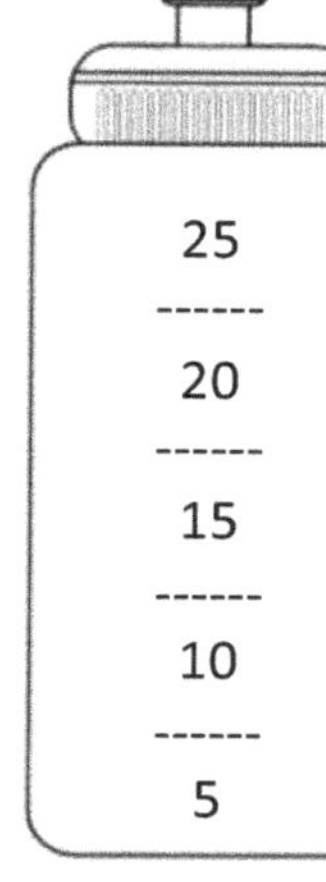
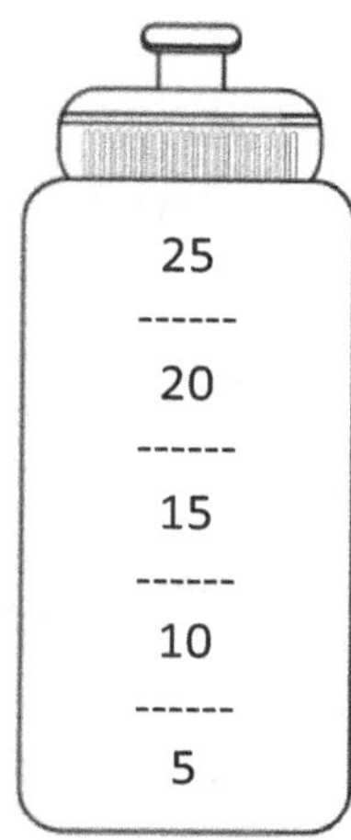

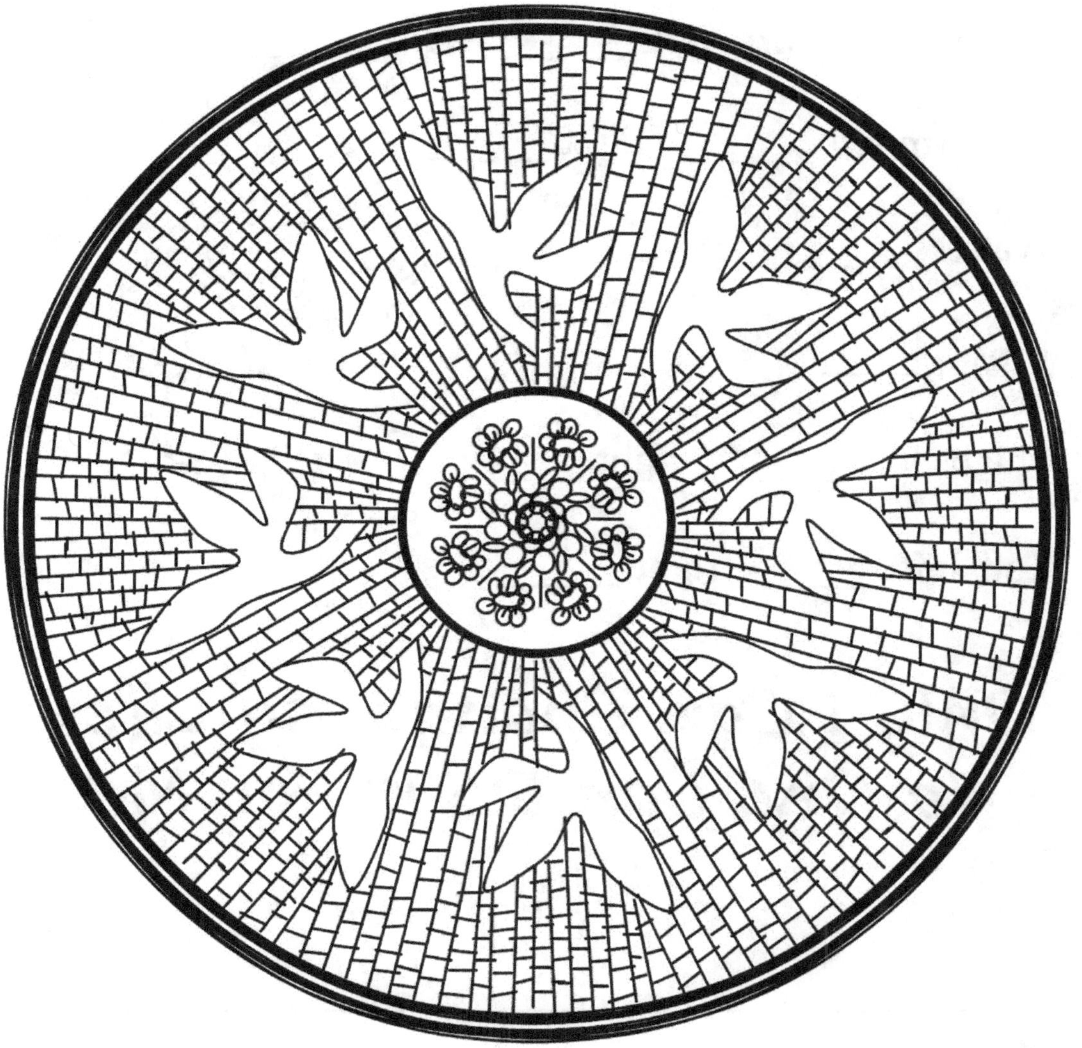

Measurements

P
R
O
G
R
E
S
S

DATE: ___________

Weight: _______

Neck _______

Shoulders _______

Chest _______

Bicep / upper arm left _________ right _______

Forearm left _________ right _______

Waist _______

Hips _______

Thighs left _______ right _______

Calf left _________ right _______

C
H
E
C
K

Only I Can Change My Life, No One Can Do It For Me!

Day Forty _______

5:00 _______________	
6:00 _______________	
7:00 _______________	_______________
8:00 _______________	_______________
9:00 _______________	_______________
10:00 ______________	_______________
11:00 ______________	
Noon _______________	**Today's victories**
1:00 _______________	
2:00 _______________	
3:00 _______________	
4:00 _______________	
5:00 _______________	
6:00 _______________	Do you believe in magic or miracles?
7:00 _______________	
8:00 _______________	_______________
9:00 _______________	_______________
10:00 ______________	_______________
11:00 ______________	_______________
Midnight ___________	_______________

The *Stella Society* Workout

Exercise	Set 1	Set 2	Set 3	Set 4	Set 5	notes

Time started: ______________   Time ended: ______________

Location: ____

Feelings before training:

Feelings after training

NUTRITION

Meal 1
time eaten: _________

Meal 2
time eaten: _________

Meal 3
time eaten: _________

Meal 4
time eaten: _________

Meal 5
time eaten: _________

Hydration

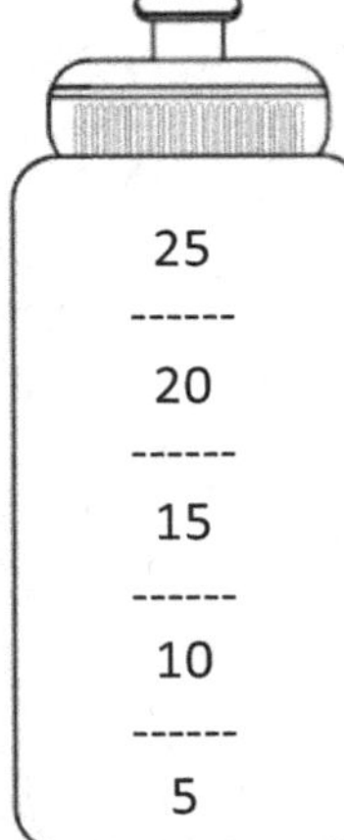
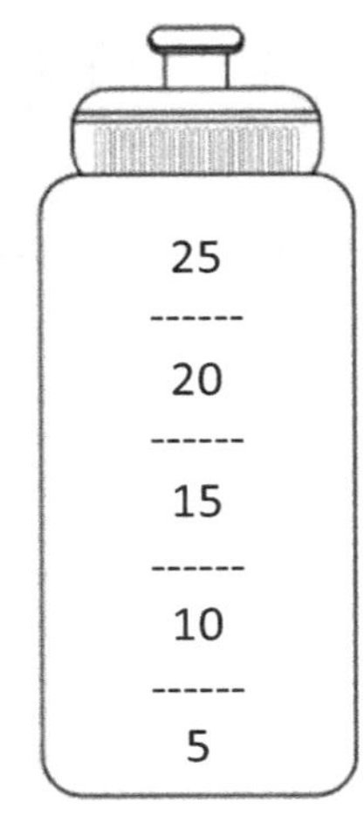
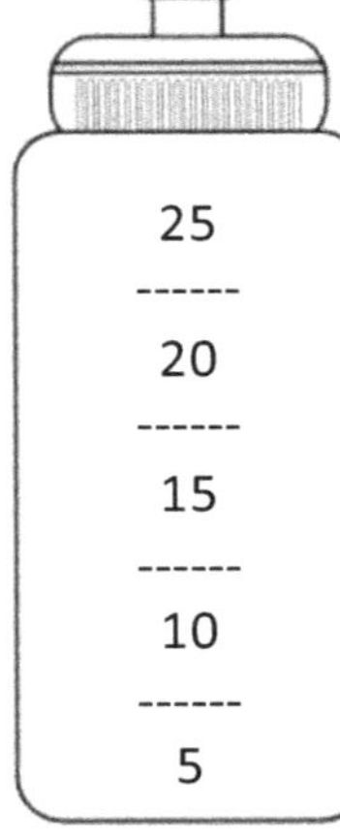
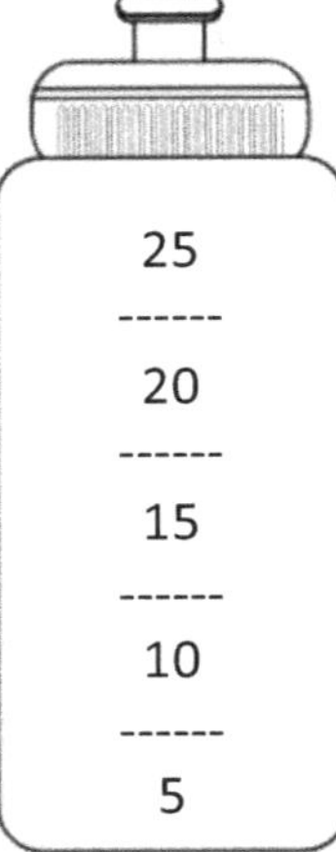
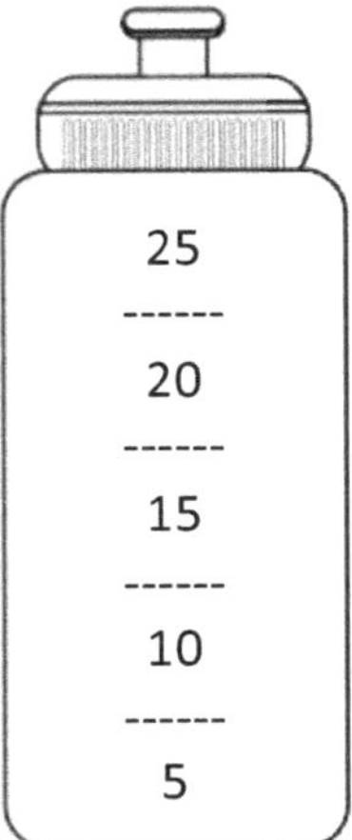

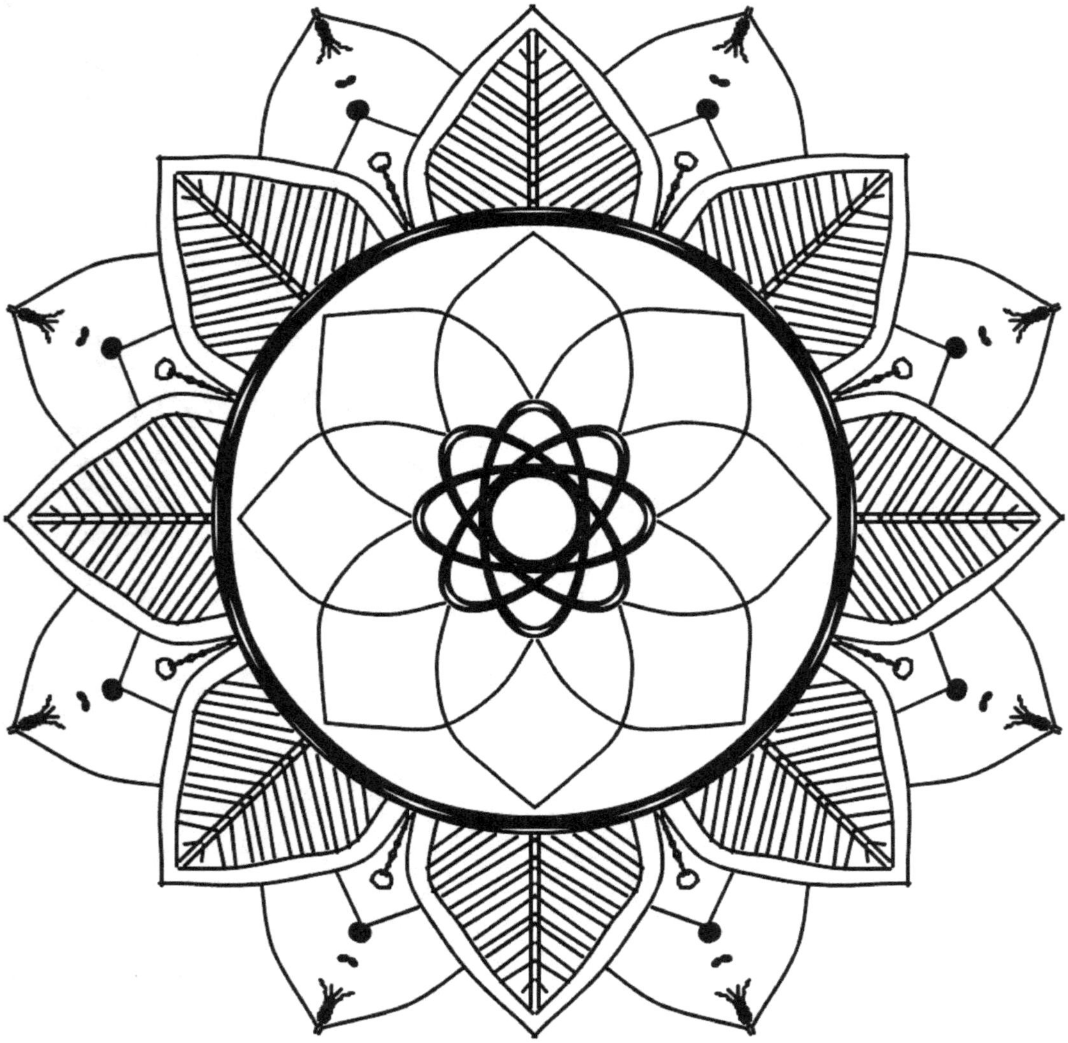

Day Forty-one ______

5:00 _________________________

6:00 _________________________

7:00 _________________________

8:00 _________________________

9:00 _________________________

10:00 _________________________

11:00 _________________________

Noon _________________________

1:00 _________________________

2:00 _________________________

3:00 _________________________

4:00 _________________________

5:00 _________________________

6:00 _________________________

7:00 _________________________

8:00 _________________________

9:00 _________________________

10:00 _________________________

11:00 _________________________

Midnight _____________________

top priorities for today

Today's victories

What is one thing you want to do forever?

The *Stella Society* Workout

Exercise	Set 1	Set 2	Set 3	Set 4	Set 5	notes

Time started: _____________ Time ended: _______________

Location: ____

Feelings before training:

Feelings after training

NUTRITION

Meal 1
time eaten: _________

Meal 2
time eaten: _________

Meal 3
time eaten: _________

Meal 4
time eaten: _________

Meal 5
time eaten: _________

Hydration

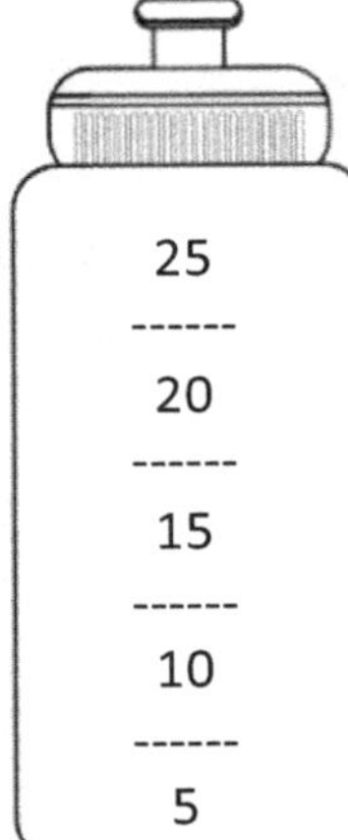

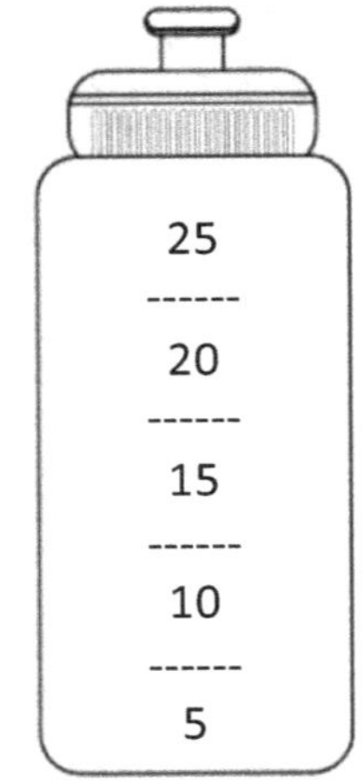

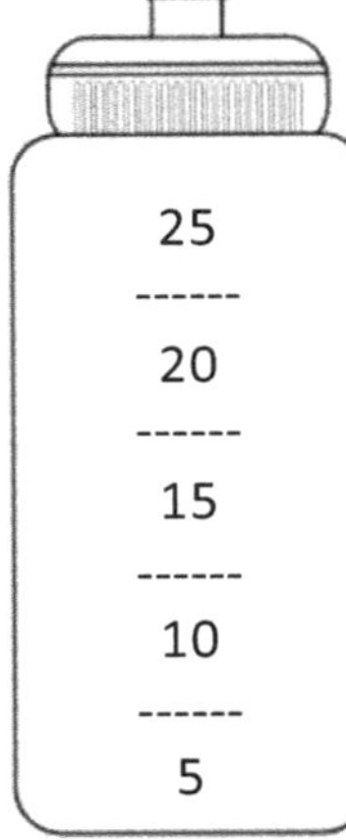

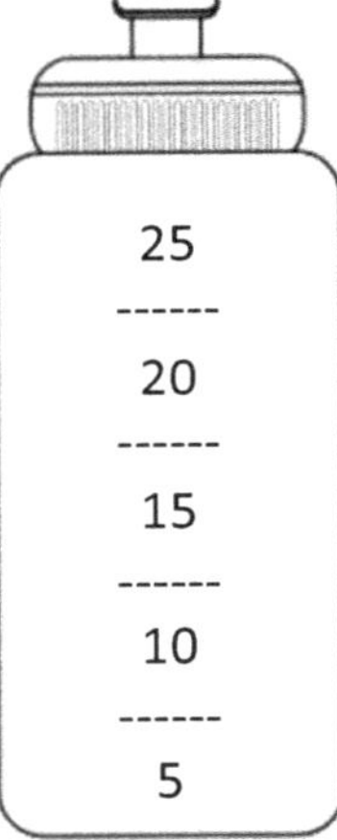

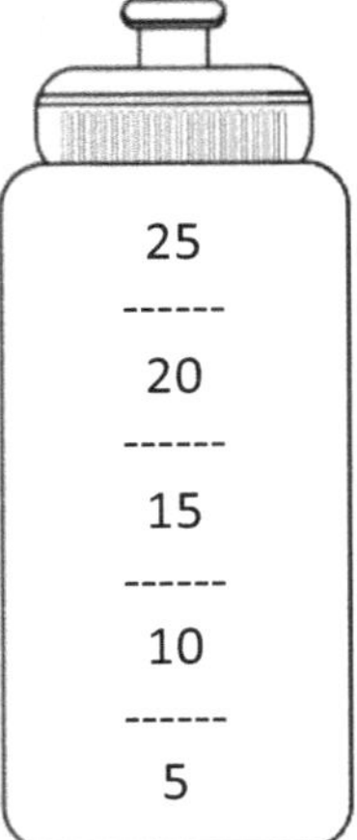

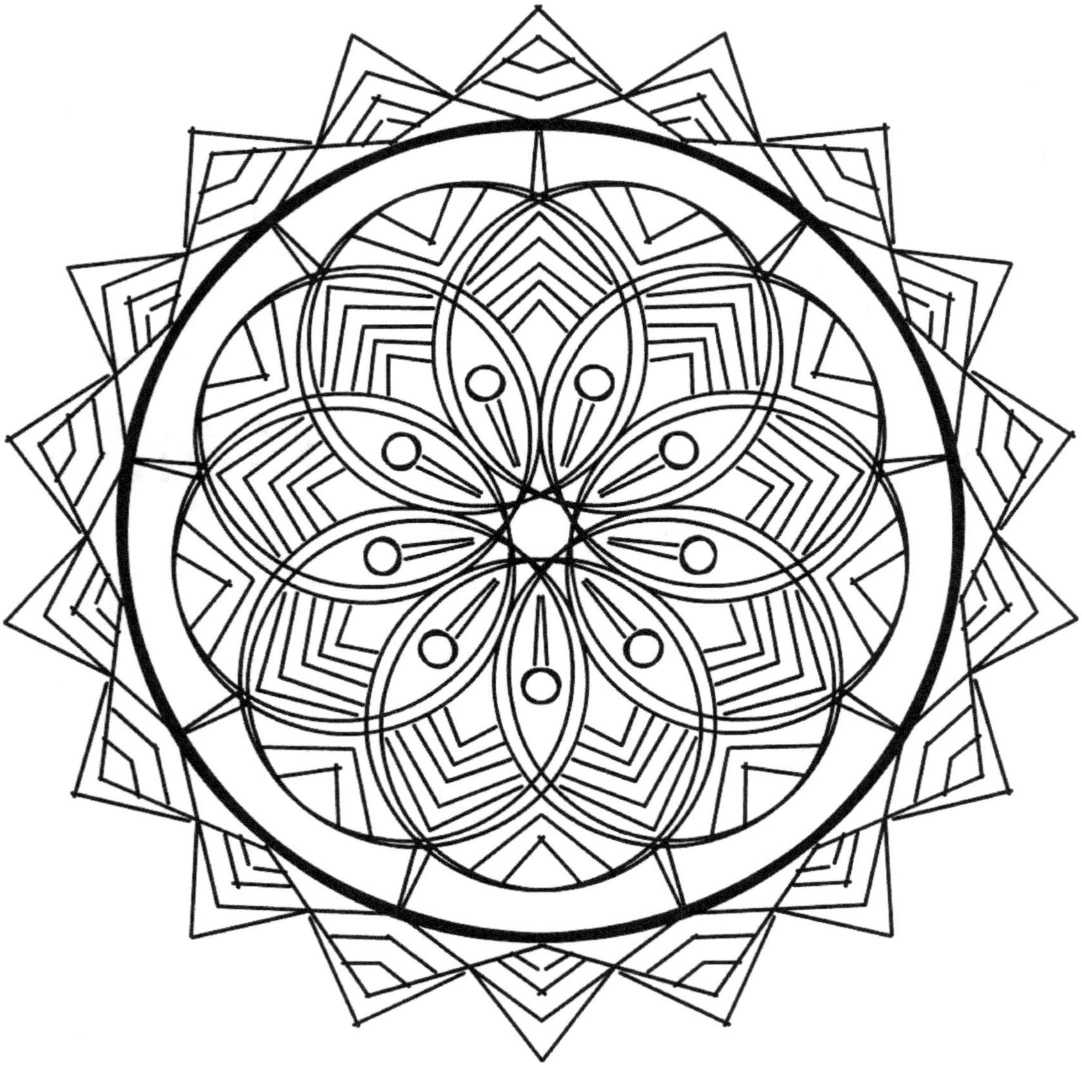

Day Forty-two _______

5:00 _______________	

____

____

____

____

Today's victories

What was your biggest
victory in the last 40 days?

____

____

____

____

____

____

____

5:00 _______________

6:00 _______________

7:00 _______________

8:00 _______________

9:00 _______________

10:00 _______________

11:00 _______________

Noon _______________

1:00 _______________

2:00 _______________

3:00 _______________

4:00 _______________

5:00 _______________

6:00 _______________

7:00 _______________

8:00 _______________

9:00 _______________

10:00 _______________

11:00 _______________

Midnight _______________

The Stella Society Workout

Exercise	Set 1	Set 2	Set 3	Set 4	Set 5	notes

Time started: _____________   Time ended: _____________

Location: ____

Feelings before training: 🙂 😐 🙁 😜 😠 😕 😊 😎

Feelings after training 🙂 😐 🙁 😜 😠 😕 😊 😎

NUTRITION

Meal 1
time eaten: _________

Meal 2
time eaten: _________

Meal 3
time eaten: _________

Meal 4
time eaten: _________

Meal 5
time eaten: _________

Hydration

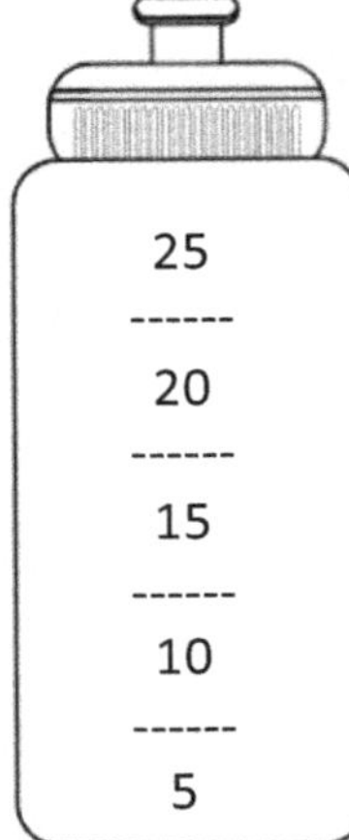
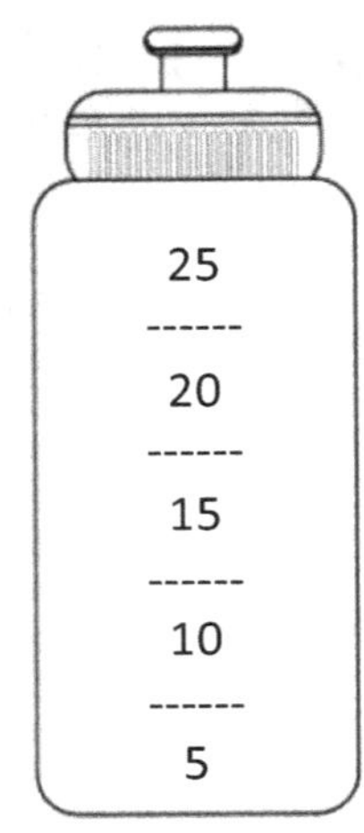
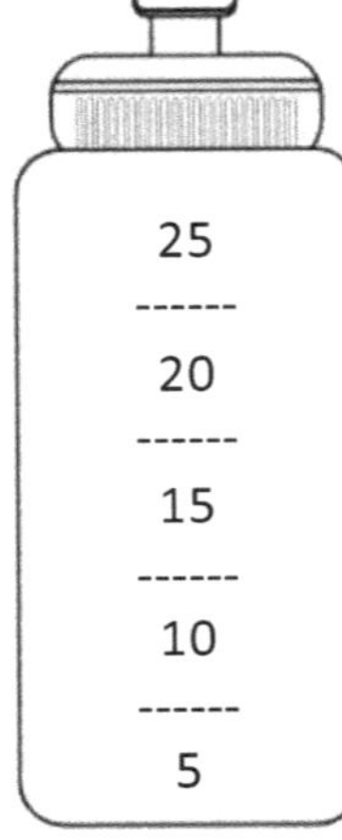
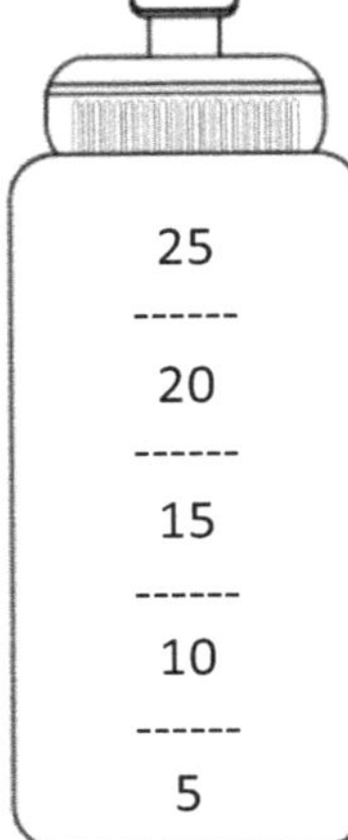
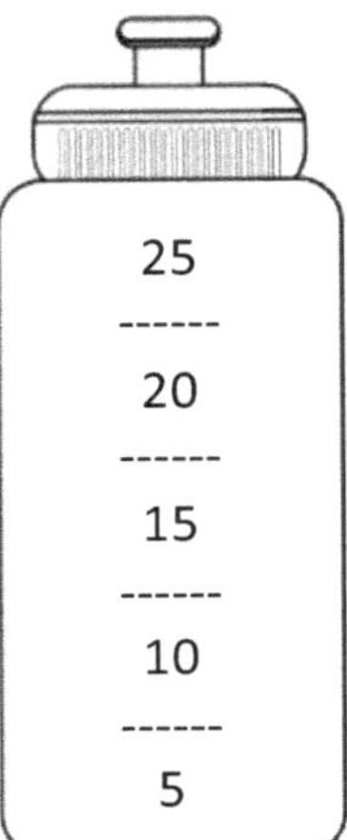

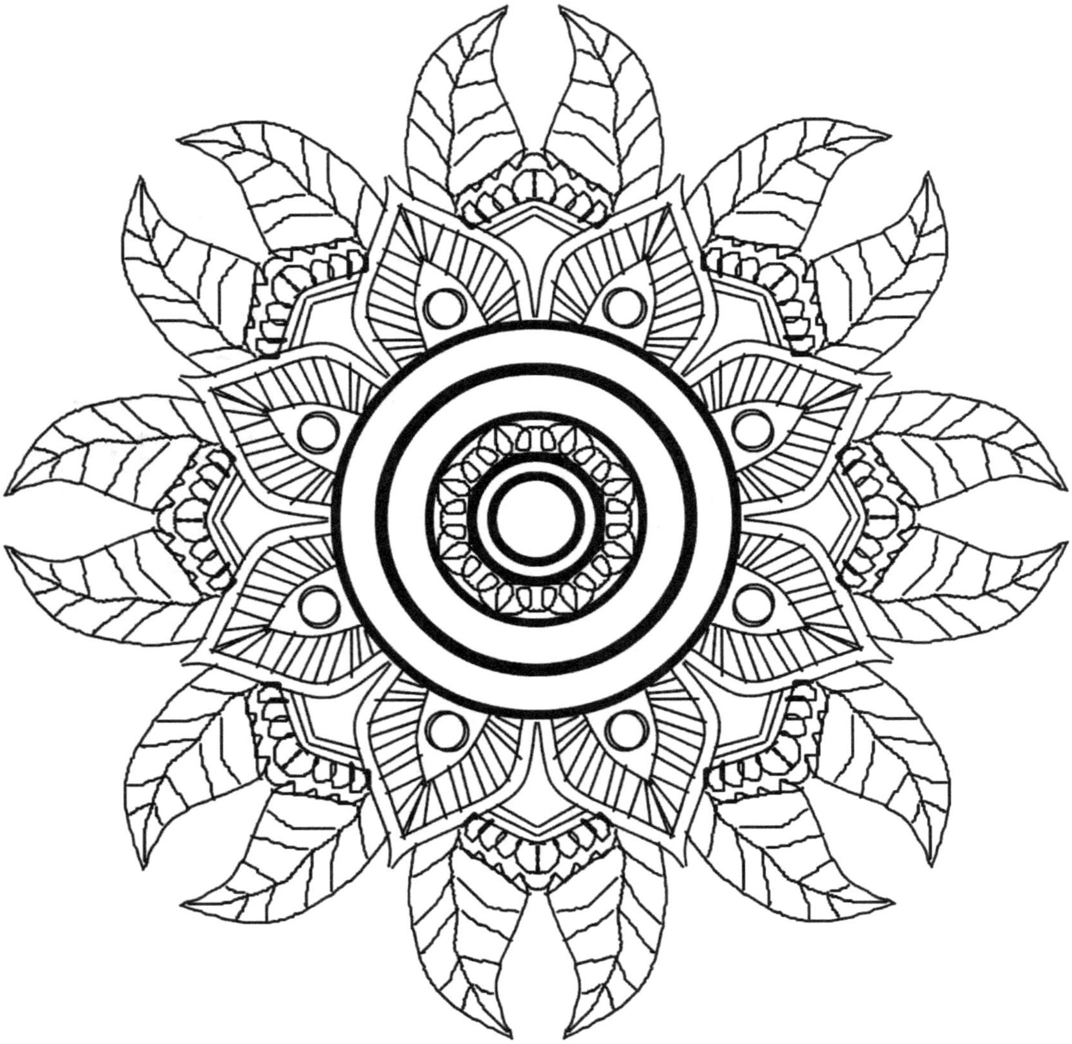

NOW WHAT?